HOW BRITAIN LOVES THE NHS
Practices of Care and Contestation

Ellen A. Stewart

P

First published in Great Britain in 2023 by

Policy Press, an imprint of
Bristol University Press
University of Bristol
1-9 Old Park Hill
Bristol
BS2 8BB
UK
t: +44 (0)117 374 6645
e: bup-info@bristol.ac.uk

Details of international sales and distribution partners are available at
policy.bristoluniversitypress.co.uk

British Library Cataloguing in Publication Data
A catalogue record for this book is available from the British Library

ISBN 978-1-4473-6887-8 paperback
ISBN 978-1-4473-6888-5 ePub
ISBN 978-1-4473-6889-2 OA PDF

Cover design: Robin Hawes
Front cover image: iStock/lubilub
Bristol University Press and Policy Press use environmentally responsible print partners.
Printed and bound in Great Britain by CPI Group (UK) Ltd, Croydon, CR0 4YY

FSC
www.fsc.org
MIX
Paper | Supporting
responsible forestry
FSC® C013604

Contents

List of figures and tables

Figures

Tables

List of abbreviations

BSAS	British Social Attitudes Survey
CSO	Chief Scientist Office (Scotland)
HF	Health Foundation
NHSCT	NHS Charities Together
PPE	Personal Protective Equipment
PPF	Public Partnership Forum
RVS	Royal Voluntary Service

Acknowledgements

I am still surprised at my boldness in writing a book about how Britain feels about anything. The title came to me while pondering the idea of a book based on my recent research. As soon as it did, I was certain it was the book I wanted to write, and everywhere I looked I saw nothing but love for the NHS. This ubiquity of grateful rhetoric about the NHS was a function of the pandemic context, which also seriously slowed my ability to write anything much beyond the title. It has taken years to get from that idea to publication and the manuscript has been completed in a period of greater contestation, amidst waves of industrial action across the NHS workforce.

Many friends and colleagues have provided encouragement to assuage the imposter syndrome which reared up in response to my boldness. Sarah Cunningham-Burley told me quite firmly that I should at least try to write another book. Kat Smith, always incisive and generous with her feedback, reviewed the proposal and helped me understand the shape of my argument. Three anonymous peer reviewers offered immensely helpful critique of the proposal and sample chapter, and another reviewed a draft of the full manuscript. The book is much better for their efforts.

Other friends, whose work has often inspired my own, have taken time to read and make insightful comments on chapters: Justyna Bandola-Gill, John Boswell, Kathy Dodworth, Thomas Elston, Colin Lorne and Fadhila Mazanderani. Both Jenny Crane and John Mohan read and commented on the whole manuscript despite many pressures on their own time. Of course, any remaining errors are entirely my own.

Much of my thinking for the book developed in the interdisciplinary space of the Wellcome Trust-funded Centre for Biomedicine, Self & Society at the University of Edinburgh. The book is very much a product of my research in dialogue with what I learnt from the sociologists, historians and ethicists who make up the Centre. I doubt I would have managed to get it written without the time and space afforded me by a move to the School of Social Work & Social Policy at the University of Strathclyde. Thanks to colleagues there for welcoming me so graciously, and for letting me get on with the work of the book before I'd done anything to prove my worth as a colleague.

Almost all of my research projects are collaborative, and much of what is reported here has been either developed or conducted with other researchers. They might not all agree with the analysis, but the following have all made valuable contributions to research reported in this book: Kathy Dodworth, Angelo Ercia, Christian Möller, Kath Bassett, Anna Nonhebel, Fadhila Mazanderani and Kayla Ostrishko. Kathy, Angelo, Chris, Kath and Anna all kindly agreed to me reproducing extracts from co-authored outputs of collaborative projects in this book.

- Sections of text in Chapter 3 are adapted from Stewart et al (2022) Doing 'Our Bit': Solidarity, Inequality, and COVID-19 Crowdfunding for the UK National Health Service, *Social Science & Medicine*, 308, reproduced under a CC by 4.0 license.
- Sections of text in Chapter 5 are adapted from Stewart, Dodworth and Ercia (2022) The Everyday Work of Hospital Campaigns: Public Knowledge and Activism in the UK's National Health Services, in Crane and Hand (Eds) *Posters, Protests and Prescriptions: Cultural Histories of the NHS in Britain*, Manchester University Press, reproduced with permission of Manchester University Press.
- Three figures in Chapter 2 (Figures 2.1, 2.2 and 2.3) are adapted from Wellings et al (2022) *Public satisfaction with the NHS and social care in 2021: results from the British Social Attitudes Survey*, with generous permission from the King's Fund and Nuffield Trust.
- The epigraph to Chapter 1 is from *The New Politics of the NHS* (seventh edition), Rudolf Klein, © 2013, CRC Press, reproduced by permission of Taylor & Francis Group.

Data reported in Figure 4.1 was shared with me by Dr Allison Smith of the Royal Voluntary Service and is adapted from Hogg and Smith (2021) *Kickstarting a New Volunteer Revolution*. The Royal Voluntary Service media team agreed to me volunteering in a café and writing about it. My manager in the café and the three volunteers whom I worked with each week were immensely kind to me, even when I proved myself quite bad at both working the till and making bacon rolls. They made the three months of volunteering a genuine pleasure.

James Munro at Care Opinion was immediately encouraging when approached about the analysis I present in Chapter 6. Care Opinion gave me a subscription to work with the data more easily, and James shared his own valuable insights with me as well as reviewing the chapter.

My sincere gratitude to the research funders who have supported the research reported here: the Economic and Social Research Council (1+3 PhD studentship at the University of Edinburgh 2007–2011), the Chief Scientist Office Scotland (postdoctoral fellowship CF/CSO/01), the Health Foundation (Policy Challenge Fund grant 7607) and, last but far from least, the Wellcome Trust (Collaborative Award 219901/Z/19/Z). Without the Wellcome Trust's willingness to support the costs of open access publishing under my Collaborative Award, not only would this book not be so widely available, but frankly I would not have written it.

Finally, of course, thanks and love to my precious family for supporting my research, and tolerating my distraction and absences while writing. Particular thanks to Sarah Stewart, who has been editing my writing for three decades, since we started writing sequels to our favourite books as children. She still hasn't fixed my dubious use of commas.

1

On loving the NHS

> An institution that often seemed to be a national problem –
> its history punctuated by crises and prophecies of impending
> collapse – has survived as a national treasure. Public support
> remains rock solid: political parties compete to proclaim their
> faith in the service and their role as guardians of its future.
>
> Klein, 2013, p 305

In Britain we often tell stories about how much we love the NHS. London's wry 2012 Olympics opening ceremony included an extravagant choreographed routine by British film director Danny Boyle. The ceremony featured (alongside James Bond, Mr Bean and Queen Elizabeth II), staff from one of Britain's most famous hospitals dancing with hospital beds on wheels which came together to spell 'NHS' in the middle of the stadium (Crane, 2019; Cowan, 2020). Popular books and television programmes centre the NHS and all its dysfunctions (Thomson, 2022). Events are held to celebrate the healthcare system's 'birthday' of 5 July (Gerada, 2021); with the 75th such birthday falling in 2023.

The volume of public feeling about the NHS was amplified during the COVID-19 pandemic, when rainbow hearts for the NHS suddenly appeared everywhere from house windows to incongruous product packaging. Clap for Carers, described in *The Guardian* as a 'very unBritish ritual' (Addley, 2020), began quite spontaneously and spread across social media as a 'nexus for thanking activities on social media' that 'became the subject of competing and conflicting notions … that were proxies for ideological battles over roles and responsibilities' (Day et al, 2022, p 159). The intensification of the NHS's cultural role during the pandemic related also to the ubiquity of NHS Charities Together's Urgent COVID-19 Appeal: corporate donations to this campaign are why mentions of the NHS appeared on everything from train displays, to drinks bottles and advent calendars in 2021.

Nonetheless societal love for the NHS was not a new phenomenon. Former Children's Laureate Michael Rosen's touching book about his hospitalisation and eventual recovery from COVID-19 is entitled *Many Different Kinds of Love: A Story of Life, Death and the NHS* (Rosen 2021), but years before COVID he wrote a poem for the 60th birthday of the NHS. In the foreword to a fundraising anthology *These Are the Hands: Poems from the Heart of the NHS*, he states that the NHS 'is at the very heart of who we are and what we are here for' (Rosen, 2020).

Researchers also tell these stories, often with a footnote or fleeting citation to Nigel Lawson's quote that 'the NHS is the closest thing the English have to a national religion'. Clarke et al (2007, p 113) reference 'a wider political and cultural significance of the NHS as the embodiment of public services in the UK'. Hannah Bradby's authoritative *Medicine, Health & Society* states that the 'enormous popular support that the NHS has from the British populace' may have repressed the development of critical, theoretically-driven medical sociology by 'constrain[ing] the range of theoretical questions about models of healthcare delivery that can be asked' (Bradby, 2012, p 8). This love is tested in opinion polls, including by national thinktanks who always seem a little bemused by the population's affection for our creaking health system. One pollster reports a research participant stating 'it is in the marrow of our bones' (Knox, 2017). These polls, as Chapter 2 will show, suggest significant and longitudinally resilient public support for the NHS. This has endured even as we have seen significant shifts in what the NHS looks like from a patient perspective, and increasing discrepancies across the four nations of the UK in the entitlements it assures.

And, of course, we show it at the ballot box. In 1952 Bevan described Churchill's Conservative Party wishing to 'kill' the new, and apparently popular, NHS: 'But they would wish it done more stealthily and in such a fashion that they would not appear to have the responsibility' (Bevan, 2010). In the New Labour era, the Conservative party's perceived negativity towards the NHS – as a canary in the mine of their wider attitudes to the UK's social safety net – seemed to render them unelectable (Klein and Rafferty, 2004; Bochel and Powell, 2018). The Conservative response to the apparently unshakeable association in voters' minds between the Labour Party and 'our' NHS has been to increase their rhetorical engagement with the NHS (Green and Hobolt, 2008; Bochel and Defty, 2010), even as they have made real terms budget cuts (Stoye, 2018; King's Fund, 2022). Reflecting Klein's (2013) quote about politicians 'compet[ing] to proclaim their faith in the service', being seen as pro-NHS remains politically important at multiple levels of governance. In an ethnographic study of local NHS politics in England, Carter and Martin described a widespread 'political reluctance to be seen to undermine the symbolic imaginary of the NHS' (Carter and Martin, 2018, p 723). The Constitution for the NHS in England begins 'the NHS belongs to us all' (NHS England, 2013), and national health policies often 'emphasise enduring national pride in the NHS' (Tuohy, 2023, p 279). In 2016, NHS England published commissioned research exploring public and stakeholder perspectives on the NHS 'brand identity', including its recognisability and its 'emotional attributes' (Research Works Limited, 2016).

As will be discussed further in Chapter 2, Britain's commitment to the NHS is also noted internationally (Berwick, 2008). Comparative health policy researcher Carolyn Tuohy describes it as 'iconically popular' (Tuohy,

2019). As will be discussed in Chapter 2, comparative survey research tends to suggest that levels of public support for the healthcare system are high in the UK. While this is in part a function of our particular, national health 'type' system (Wendt et al, 2010; Jordan, 2013), this is, at the very least, a story that Britain enjoys telling about itself. This generates a kind of self-reinforcing cultural mystique which can seem increasingly divorced from the nuts and bolts of healthcare delivery. For Tuohy, this embedded institutional narrative is of 'the NHS as a proud national achievement, founded in adversity and faithfully preserved through periodic peril by its dedicated staff as a single institution, publicly accountable to citizens and providing comprehensive healthcare, universal and free at the point of service' (Tuohy, 2023, p 294).

The driving force behind this book is a sense that Britain's 'love' for the NHS is stated too often but examined too rarely, and often too superficially. Public support for the NHS is, in academic research, often a backdrop against which the 'real' business of health politics is described playing out. But the everyday experiences through which members of the public encounter the NHS – as patients, carers, staff, taxpayers and community members – are rich, complex, and as worthy of proper attention as the power politics of Westminster. Building on a decade of empirical research on publics within the NHS, I argue that the compulsion to declare, and reluctance to interrogate, public commitment to the NHS glosses over some profound conflicts and societal fissures. I propose another way to understand and 'know' how we love the NHS, going beyond the rhetorical or declarative to explore the practices through which we encounter, and value it. These practices, I argue, should be understood as not merely communicating love for the NHS, but enacting it through care, and by actively contesting its future. To conclude the book, I explore some of the more dysfunctional consequences of the way we have approached public love for the NHS, and propose that understanding these sentiments as more complex and multi-dimensional phenomena, offers a more generative way forward.

Loving the NHS, past and present

This book is about how Britain loves the NHS now, in the second decade of the 21st century and the long end stages of the COVID-19 pandemic. Chapters explore practices from between the early 2010s and 2022. But it contributes to a long, sometimes cluttered catalogue of studies of the NHS in which public support looms large. In 2008 Marmor described the NHS as 'a lightning rod for health policy commentary' (Marmor, 2008, p 329). The same year, Gorsky (2008, p 438) reviewed the historiography of the NHS as 'at once small and manageable, and vast and unwieldy'. While the book is about 'now', I am mindful both that 'now' is imbued with the decades that came before it, and that 'now' will very quickly be, itself, history. I do not attempt to review the decades of commentary and scholarship which have chronicled our health system's development – Gorsky's (2008) authoritative and clear-sighted essay will help readers seeking that – but contemporary studies of social and public policies require better engagement with what came before (Lewis, Gewirtz and Clarke, 2000).

The history of the NHS is conventionally told chronologically, often as a series of sequential crises or 'transformations' (Gorsky, 2008; Klein, 2013). Within these, public support for the NHS is generally stated, but rarely closely examined. Klein's (2013) influential history of the organisation of the NHS argues that over the decades, and accelerating during the New Labour reforms, the NHS has shifted from paternalistic 'church' to a consumeristic 'garage'. This is identified as an 'over-arching narrative' (Gorsky, 2008, p 441) of NHS scholarship. Despite the central role attributed here to public and patient roles (as faithful congregation or assertive consumers), Klein's exposition of the two models is intrinsically top down, and based on an account of policy discourse and tools, not of public feeling. One reviewer notes this omission: commenting that the book offers a sophisticated and commanding history of health policy in the NHS, and not of popular health politics (Brown, 2015). Klein acknowledges that the 'church to garage' story is a simplification (Klein, 2010), and indeed the parsimony of his accounts are widely considered to be crucial to his contribution to the complexity of the NHS (Helderman, 2015). However, some of the standard narratives of the NHS as national achievement have been subject to a number of more substantive reassessments.

One key critique is a scholarly reappraisal of what Millar (2022) describes as the NHS's 'origin story'. This story relies upon a vaunted 'spirit of '45', presented as a moment of startling and productive solidarity following the 'total war' that had come before (Lowe, 1990; Harris, 2004), seeding the creation of the NHS in 1948 (Bivins, 2020). Stanley describes this as 'a founding myth to *post-imperial* Britishness' (Stanley, 2022, p 18). The NHS, then, is beloved because it represents solidarity, borne of suffering, and nostalgia. Postcolonial scholars have identified the near total neglect, within this conventional narrative, of the manner in which Britain's welfare state, its 'gift' to the populace who had served and suffered, was made possible by both the financial legacy of Britain's empire, and its ongoing exploitation via Commonwealth recruitment of staff (Bhambra, 2022a; Hansen, 2022). The NHS, then, should be seen as 'an imperially resourced public service' (Fitzgerald et al, 2020, p 1161) and we must recognise the 'cognitive dissonance' of celebrations of the NHS as a progressive British achievement which exclude the violently repressive imperial work which made it possible (Meer, 2022).

As well as troubling more rose-tinted visions of public spiritedness in the early years of the NHS, historians who have focused more explicitly and substantively on public feeling for the NHS describe a more chequered trajectory of sentiment beyond 1948. Arnold-Forster and Gainty (2021) describe a lukewarm reception from patients in the service's early years. Seaton (2015) chronicles continued overt opposition to Britain's 'sacred cow', albeit led by doctors rather than members of the public. To some extent, the idea of universal public love for the NHS across the population almost inevitably crumbles under scrutiny. But histories of the NHS also posit that a more assertively supportive public attitude emerged as a key artefact of decisions taken in the 1980s and 1990s, including proactive NHS branding in the aftermath of internal market reforms (Bivins, 2015; Thomson, 2022). Crane (2019) argues that public activism around the NHS – 'campaigning explicitly about the NHS, as a whole' was an innovation forged in the contentious context of 1980s politics. In this way, the intensification of feeling around the NHS that we saw during the COVID-19 pandemic can be seen as the culmination of political strategies with much longer roots.

What can we learn from these dominant narratives of how Britain has loved the NHS since its creation, and their reappraisals? First, they suggest that the binary models of the NHS as church or garage have value, but many omissions (a point which Klein himself makes in his original essay). Simplifications such as 'the state's role in medical care has shifted from an expression of social solidarity and public service to a means of satisfying the preferences of increasingly "autonomous" patients' (Gorsky, 2008, p 441) have broad brush value. Helderman (2015) argues that Klein's books offer up a valuable 'collective memory' of the NHS, and hint that they might not merely chronicle, but sustain it:

> Collective memories not only remind us of where we came from, they also remind us of what we consider to be important values that we should care for and that we (wish to) share and sustain with other members of the collectivity. Collective memories contribute to the establishment of moral and ethical norms in defence of universal and impartial political institutions, such as the NHS. (Helderman, 2015, p 229)

Because collective memories have consequences, it is vital that stories we tell ourselves about public sentiment acknowledge conflicting experiences and views. The rainbow love hearts that sprang up during the early months of the pandemic, when a relatively small proportion of the population were actively seeking or receiving patient care, don't preclude a broader shift to consumerism, but nor do they reveal a resurgence of an uncomplicated solidaristic fervour across the population.

Second, we must attend more, and better, to the exclusions contained within contemporary celebrations of the NHS. What kind of healthcare are we celebrating when we stand, clapping on our doorsteps amid a pandemic? Bhambra's (2022b, p 13) characterisation of 'the web of reciprocity in which obligations are recognized' is mobilised specifically to highlight colonial exclusions from and exploitations within the claimed beneficence of the welfare state, but could also be applied to other groups, inside and outside the UK. At the height of the pandemic, Gary Younge (2020) wrote a moving column about his personal associations with the NHS, and the ambivalence with which he celebrated it during 'clap for carers':

> I am clapping for the NHS and the people who work in it, as my mother did; for the disproportionately black and brown migrant and low-paid labourers who keep the institution going, have done so since its inception and are now disproportionately vulnerable to both the disease and lockdown's challenges. I'm clapping with pride that I live in a nation that has created and sustained this, but also with rage that they still do not all have the protective equipment or testing they need, and with hope that one day soon they'll get the pay they deserve and the service the investment it needs. (Younge, 2020)

As well as being predominantly top-down (Gorsky, 2008), the NHS's discursive history has been told overwhelmingly by white male academics. Rather than a singular account of how the population feels about the NHS, this book seeks, however imperfectly, to draw together the narratives of a wider group, including those 'left out of its formal narration' (Meer, 2022), to offer a more complex picture *within* the context of this favoured national story.

What is this thing we call the NHS?

A book about how Britain loves the NHS must, at a baseline, offer a coherent account of the object of that love. Yet on even the lightest of examinations, the ontology of the NHS is replete with contradictions. Is the NHS in the 21st century an idea, a promise, a set of buildings and services? Is it its staff, its patients and the officials who, for more than 70 years, have been trying to manage it? What role does the NHS 'brand' – the colour, the logo, the websites – that NHS England (2022c) explicitly describes as one of the most 'cherished and recognised brands in the world' play in our sense of what it *is*?

My previous research, and that of sociologists interested in healthcare architecture and design, has suggested that public feeling about the NHS is often significantly focused on the 'bricks and mortar' of healthcare, specifically hospitals (Martin et al, 2015; Stewart, 2019). While this might seem a robust object for affection, in practice the 'NHS estate', as it is described in policy terms (Nuffield Trust, 2018), is permanently in flux

(Fulop et al, 2012; Jones, Fraser and Stewart, 2019). Hospitals and beds close, with the number of hospital beds in England alone halving between 1988 and 2019 (Ewbank et al, 2021). Many ostensibly NHS hospitals are built, owned and managed by private companies, and only leased to the NHS (Hellowell and Pollock, 2009). But beyond that, NHS hospitals are moved to new sites, extended, rebuilt and refurbished. Indeed, as digital healthcare becomes mainstream, physical buildings might recede within the set of infrastructures that make up a health system. Enhanced provision of digital care means that in the last two years, many of us have mostly encountered the NHS in our homes (Langstrup, 2013), at the other end of a telephone or video call (Hutchings, 2020). So, while there is plenty of evidence that the British public cares *about* NHS buildings, those buildings are changing in makeup and relevance, much more than our apparently steady affection for our health system.

If our NHS buildings are less permanent than sometimes assumed, perhaps Britain's love for the NHS is oriented towards the people who staff our NHS (Saunders, 2022). Especially during the COVID-19 pandemic, NHS staff were often recast and lauded as 'our NHS heroes'. On Thursday evenings in the early months of the pandemic the 'clap for carers' celebrated the sacrifice of NHS staff and other keyworkers on doorsteps across Britain. This ostensible moment of unity should not be overstated: 'We clearly aren't all clapping for the same thing' (Younge, 2020). It is also significant that such 'heroic' narratives can stifle criticism of unsafe working conditions, and normalise levels of personal risk for which healthcare professionals had never signed up (Cox, 2020; Mohammed et al, 2021). Staff wellbeing was one of the key goals of NHS Charities Together's highly successful fundraising campaign (to be discussed further in Chapter 3). During this, companies sought to be associated with 'one of the most cherished and recognised brands in the world' (NHS England, 2022c), and members of the public signed up to 'do their bit' for our NHS heroes.

Gratitude and affection for NHS staff are grounded in, and even increased by acknowledgement of their often-challenging working environments. A 2021 report identified 'chronic excessive workloads' as underlying poor health and retention within the workforce in England, as well as creating an impossible 'vicious circle of staff shortages and excessive workload that is the most cited reason for staff leaving health and social care organisations' (Bailey and West, 2021). These workforce gaps have long been plugged by enthusiastic recruitment of health professionals first from the Commonwealth and then from a wider range of low and middle income countries (Kyriakides and Virdee, 2003; Bivins, 2015). There is longstanding evidence that the medical workforce experiences racism in the NHS (Kyriakides and Virdee, 2003; Woodhead et al, 2022). And the 'hostile environment' migration policies pursued in recent years have only exacerbated these experiences: some of the most painful tales from the 'Windrush scandal' in which people resident in the UK for decades were detained and in some cases deported due to new immigration policies, concerned people who had taken up invitations to the UK to staff the NHS (Williams, 2020).

The conceptual apparatus through which we perceive the NHS does not help us define an object of all this love. The NHS clearly is not and never has been a singular organisation, but a system of healthcare, connoting not merely linked organisations of delivery but a wider range of actors, values and relationships (Kielmann, Hutchinson and MacGregor, 2022). The ways in which the NHS is a system are, though, rarely theorised (Freeman and Frisina, 2010). And sometimes smaller units within it (at national, regional or even local levels) declare *themselves* to be systems. In England the organisations which make up this system have been repeatedly fragmented, brought together again under curious umbrellas, and redivided by policy reforms (Smith, Walshe and Hunter, 2001), most recently into Integrated Care Systems. In 2023 Scotland, Northern Ireland and Wales all demonstrate a more 'classical' NHS structure, in which unelected managers, accountable to central government, lead NHS organisations responsible for most of the services across a defined geographical area. These differences are frequently overlooked in England (McHale et al, 2021), but are increasingly altering the experience of healthcare in the devolved nations.

Living and working in Scotland, I have spent much of my academic career politely correcting scholars who research the NHS in England and refer to it simply as 'the NHS', eliding and erasing the significant differences across the UK's constituent nations (Smith and Hellowell, 2012; Greer, 2016). And so it feels incongruous for me, specifically, to be publishing a book which centres 'the NHS' as a unitary entity. Doing so is neither laziness, nor ignorance about the differences between health policy in the four nations. Rather it is a recognition that in popular and cultural discourses, 'the NHS' that we talk about, represent and 'love' has become significantly decoupled from the material realities of buildings, people and organisations. In a survey of NHS activists, Crane (2022) notes that their narratives centred 'a vision of the NHS as an abstract ideal, rather than as a system of primary, secondary, and community care settings', with a specific focus on universal access to healthcare. Sally Sheard (2022) recently wrote a poignant, thoughtful essay arguing that 'I'm afraid, there is no NHS'. I have significant respect for the line of argument, and especially for Sheard's reflections on some of the affective baggage of making such a statement. Even retyping the words feels difficult; my own affective response to what Freeman (2008) describes as the NHS's 'existential significance' is inevitably present as I write.

However this book makes a slightly different argument, inspired especially by Shona Hunter's (2016) account of the NHS as 'an affective formation'.

I argue that the NHS still exists, but in multiple: highly variegated, and perhaps even significantly depleted processes and organisations delivering healthcare across the UK, *and* as an imagined symbolic entity at a UK level. Cowan (2021), in an effort to get hold of the NHS analytically, follows a single patient pathway (hip replacement) to trace the assemblage from the bottom up. She explains: 'By following these lines of thought, I found that the NHS is no longer then a fetishized symbol, centred in the middle of the room, but something that continually gets made in heterogenous ways by everyday practices, including those made by researchers themselves.' In the chapter which proposes the concept of the NHS as an affective formation, Hunter (2016), appropriately, from an empirical point of view, specifies the English NHS as the titular affective formation of her analysis. In my view, even those of us well-attuned to the differences that have followed (and to a lesser extent, predated) devolution recognise that there is an imagined 'NHS' at UK level, even as its constituent organisations diverge. Significantly, and following Painter (2006), imagined does not in this context mean illusory: 'Social imaginaries can have very real effects' (Painter, 2006).

An approach which takes seriously the cultural and the affective requires a shift in orientation from the studies of straightforward public opinion described in Chapter 2 towards a more dynamic and reflexive understanding of the NHS as object. As Elkind (1998, p 1715) wrote, describing the value of metaphoric thinking in understanding the NHS: 'Our ability to achieve a comprehensive "reading" of a complex and ambiguous phenomenon depends on being able to see how different aspects of it may co-exist in a complementary or even paradoxical way.' As an object of public love, the NHS as symbolic entity is closely associated with its visual branding; the characteristic 'NHS blue' and the logo. Thomson (2021) identifies these as an artefact of the late 1990s, as the then New Labour government undertook a 'self-conscious branding exercise' in the face of the complexities involved in the still new internal market. *What* it symbolises is harder to identify. Is public love, far from Klein's (2010) assertion that it has become conditional, cautious, consumeristic, in fact thriving and attached to symbolism of the founding principles of the NHS (themselves frequently contested [Ruane, 1997]): universal, comprehensive and free at the point of use, funded by general taxation? This ambivalence about the ontology of the NHS explains my focus on *how* Britain loves the NHS, and not merely how *much* it does so. This book requires us to hold onto a sense of the NHS as multiple. Its different manifestations – including embodied episodes of care, documents, buildings – do not make up a single entity, like parts of a machine (Elkind, 1998), but instead exist in parallel. Like other troublesome concepts, notably the state (Painter, 2006) these components are shifting and impermanent, but are nonetheless consequential for us both individually and as a society.

Why love? Satisfaction, attitudes and experiences

The choice to centre this book on love is also a deliberate one. It stems from a conviction that the way we talk about the NHS in the UK is more affective than is suggested by wider literatures on either consumer satisfaction with healthcare or public attitudes to welfare. Crane identifies the way that NHS campaigners from the 1980s centred 'love' in free text responses to a survey despite questions avoiding the term (Crane, 2022). This is a deliberate turn towards collective affect beyond the calculated evaluations of individual satisfaction (Wendt et al, 2011). Much of the academic scholarship on 'love' is focused on romantic love, or less often familial love (Rogers and Robinson, 2014), but this book is about societal love. Affect theory distinguish emotions from sentiments, and the love I am exploring is best captured in the latter term, defined as: 'Trans-situational, generalized affective responses to specific symbols in a culture ... more socially-constructed and enduring than emotional responses' (Rogers and Robinson, 2014). That is, I argue not that every individual in Britain loves all their experiences with the NHS (as will be discussed especially in Chapter 6), but that a deeply affective view of our health system exists on a generalised level.

In understanding the dimensions of love for the NHS, we can learn from a wealth of sophisticated research which examines citizens' attitudes to the welfare state more generally. There is an especially longstanding vein of research on attitudes to social security benefits. This is a mainstay of social policy research, identifying that public attitudes to the welfare state are not a quickfire stimulus and reaction to current political decisions, but are shaped by much broader 'welfare regimes' where different 'families' of welfare states share underpinning and influential social structures (Bambra, 2005b; Freeman and Frisina, 2010). More recent branches of this scholarship also identify that discursive narratives about welfare *recipients* – as deserving, or as scroungers – can be escalated by popular media (Jensen, 2014), and even by defensive 'othering' from welfare recipients themselves (Garthwaite, 2016). Social policy researchers have demonstrated the extent to which publics misconstrue who gains from the welfare state, routinely imagining themselves to be poorer and less well-supported than they are (Greve 2022; Hills, 2017). Healthcare generally (Wendt et al, 2011), and British attitudes towards the NHS specifically (Bambra, 2005b), have been noted as anomalous outliers within wider welfare structures. That is, the NHS displays profoundly different logics from the wider British welfare state (Bambra, 2005b): considered along with Canadian Medicare, examples of 'universal programs in otherwise targeted welfare states' (Jordan, 2013).

However a more complex academic literature conceptualising *how* the population values, and imagines its benefits from, health systems has not emerged. Social policy scholars have employed an ever broader and more creative range of methods to understand public attitudes to welfare embedded in everyday life (Garthwaite, 2016; Hitchen and Raynor, 2020; Holmes and Hall, 2020; Jupp, 2022). When it comes to public attitudes to healthcare – to welfare state provision of care rather than of money – academic scholarship has been more limited (Daly and Lewis, 2000), and less creative. As discussed more in Chapter 2, Burlacu and Roescu (2021) identify three distinct literatures surveying members of the public on: their degree of (normative) solidarity; their satisfaction with health services received; and the degree to which healthcare is a salient health politics issue. They conclude that these literatures have been 'almost completely disarticulated' from each other.

Beyond the enumeration of patient satisfaction across health systems, one area where we have an overwhelming amount of high quality detailed research, is in exploring *patient* experiences of using healthcare services, and at times these stand in for 'lay' appreciations (Pols, 2005) of the wider health system. To render that intimate, personal experience on a grander scale such studies inevitably need to focus tightly on one intervention, or treatment, or perhaps health condition. Medical sociology and health services research allow us to better understand and refine the delivery of medical care. They produce lots of knowledge about a single intervention, and how it could be improved in different contexts (Davies, 2003). But they pay scant attention to an alternative dimension of how the wider population values a health system: 'Studies on public support towards healthcare systems often do not clearly distinguish between preferences regarding the role of the state in healthcare provision and the level of satisfaction with healthcare systems' (Wendt et al, 2010).

Burlacu and Roescu (2021) describe this as a blurring of the evaluative and the normative within some survey research on attitudes to healthcare. When satisfaction with care received is conflated with wider valuation of healthcare, the primary status from which we might know and value a health system becomes that of 'patient', and space for more other-regarding solidaristic sentiment is reduced. For many, this will be a fleeting identity, which does not endure beyond episodic experiences of care, making it curious to talk of a stable 'patient perspective' (Pols, 2005). However even where patienthood becomes an enduring identity, often based on long-term, chronic conditions and profound suffering (Gilbert, 2014), it is not the totality of how we encounter our health system.

If, as I have argued, there is a gap between our knowledge of how we value the NHS as patients, and how we value the NHS as citizens, from what other subject positions might we explore public affection towards the NHS? In research on the (then) emergent position of the 'citizen-consumer' in British public services, Clarke et al (2007) identified the particularity of how people talk about their position in the NHS, as compared to other services (including policing and social care), and especially the strong commitment to 'patient', and rejection of 'consumer', as descriptors. Overall, this research did not identify a straightforward shift to consumerism within British debates on healthcare. Despite its association as 'the most professionally or medically defined identity' their interviewees and focus group participants held firmly to the language of patienthood: as one put it 'no fancy or alternative word is necessary'; another described the term service user as 'politically correct psychobabble' (Clarke et al, 2007, p 130). The research emphasised though that a preference to be identified as a patient does not, in this context, imply passivity or a conventional Parsonian 'sick role' (Parsons, 1951). Clarke et al identified a particular and complex reading of patienthood within the UK health system, in which close relationship with a doctor was valued within the context of a broader commitment to (and willingness to sacrifice for) the health system as 'a collective, inclusive public resource'. They conclude that 'as a result we may need to think that the NHS is always a double entity – both a specific assemblage of organisations, people, practices and an idea, an ideal, or a representation' (Clarke et al, 2007).

This multiplicity is inherent within my approach, which seeks to find a position in which we can see the health system as the site of both deeply personal, embodied experiences, and as a site of communal identity and contestation (Sturdy, 2002). The sensitivity and nuance with which medical sociologists explore patient experience is part of the story of the health system, too easily ignored by political scientists. Yet the organisational and political structures which shape those experiences are a key frame for these stories, often treated too lightly in health services and applied medical sociology research (Davies, 2003).

This book's approach: towards a sociology of public love for the NHS

This book, then, tries to balance this multiplicity to offer an account of a healthcare *system* as it intervenes into the most intimate aspects of people's lives, and as a *public good*, with the widest of systemic consequences. I argue that the UK displays a degree of societal affection for the NHS which is reasonably resilient to individual patient experience. I attribute this to the still unusual degree of centralised state control of healthcare in the UK (Or et al, 2010) which causes heightened political visibility of health policy in the UK, as compared to other countries (Weale, 2015). Decisions and experiences that would stay local in many health systems escalate to the national stage more frequently here (Stewart et al, 2020). Less attention has been paid to the mechanisms of this visibility. Rather than an episodic flurry of interest in the NHS, when a bad news story or critical report hits the headlines, this book suggests that such events tap into a deeper, ongoing reservoir of public care for the health system. This means that community support scaffolds organisations under immense pressure to meet increasing health needs within a constrained budget envelope (Jupp, 2022). It also means that, even when the NHS fails individuals and (more problematically) systematically fails specific groups within society along lines of gender, ethnicity or (dis)ability, the sentiment of public love for the NHS endures. Loving the NHS in general can be significantly decoupled from experiences of harm and indignity which might take place within it.

I approach this societal sentiment by following and exploring a series of public practices focused on the NHS. As Chapter 2 will demonstrate, the dominant knowledge on which we base claims about Britain's love for the NHS comes from opinion polls. These answers given, often quickly, to a closed survey question, have some real value. They should allow us to identify demographic differences in how groups within the poll sample respond differently to questions about the NHS. Do people of different ethnicities express their love for the NHS differently from White British respondents? Do younger people value the NHS less, more or much the same as older people? Significantly, these polls can also offer a longitudinal picture of public opinion, showing, for example, how affection for the NHS might be expressed differently before, during and after the COVID-19 pandemic. Once these numbers have been analysed, checked and turned into colourful graphs, tables and infographics, they have a life of their own, detached from the people who gave the answers and with all ambivalence, uncertainty or second thoughts excised. I have sat through multiple presentations where researchers announce these numbers, and then we discuss whether this quantified opinion is an asset to UK healthcare or an anomalous obstacle to its transformation.

These numbers can thus give us a sense of how much Britain loves the NHS. What they can't give us is a deeper picture of the complexity behind the ticked box on a survey, nor its ambivalence, nor its political consequences (Dallinger, 2022). This is the terrain of qualitative research, which relies on a range of methods including interviews, observations and analyses of written and visual sources. These tend to offer fuller and more nuanced accounts of smaller sections or sub-groups of the population, in which people's expressed views are understood in their social and material context, rather than extracted and standardised into numerical form. These types of knowledge are foundational to how sociologists in particular have studied people's experiences of healthcare in the UK. But this book is grounded in the belief that we need to understand both societal relationships with the NHS as a health system and how people feel about their own experiences of care. This means that the tools we use to understand 'customer satisfaction' or even the less consumeristic 'patient experience' will not, alone, answer the question of how Britain loves the NHS.

This book takes a different approach in search of the more mundane or 'everyday' terrain of societal sentiment (Jupp, 2022). In an effort to open up a more expansive and multi-faceted answer to the question of how Britain loves the NHS I explore a series of meaningful social practices: campaigning, donating time or money and 'making do' when using services. Meaningful social practices here are understood as repertoires of actions which can be understood as an entity, but which are generally observed only through specific performances of that practice in context (Maller, 2015). For example, Chapter 4 of this book explores 'volunteering' as an NHS practice, by investigating particular performances of voluntarism in the contemporary NHS. One advantage to centring practices, rather than verbal statements of opinion or attitude, is that it makes space for the unspoken. This is one route to understanding societal sentiments that 'cannot be reduced to calculability, intentionality and responsibility … they can be enacted without subjects being able to articulate reasons' (Isin, 2009). While especially helpful when attempting to access knowledge held by actors who are unable to verbally articulate the reasons for their preferences (Pols, 2005), researching practices also contextualises the artificiality of asking people to state their opinions on something they may rarely explicitly consider (Eliasoph, 1998). Importantly, these social practices are understood as involving both care for the healthcare system, and contestation about its future.

Conclusion

The book proceeds as follows. Chapter 2 reviews what public opinion research tells us about public views on the NHS, but also considers where this data comes from, and what role it plays in UK media and policy discourse. The following chapters present empirical analyses of four different sets of practices through which publics interact with the NHS: fundraising money; volunteering; and campaigning. In Chapter 6, I present an analysis of patient feedback on emergency care to explore how views on the NHS suffuse patients' descriptions of experiences of care. In Chapter 7, I build on the empirical chapters to propose an over-arching conceptualisation of how Britain loves the NHS, drawing on Hunter's account of the NHS as 'affective formation' (Hunter, 2016). Seeking to move beyond critical takes which dismiss public affection for the NHS as simply irrational, or indeed as nothing more than nostalgia for an imagined and monocultural welfare state that never was, I also ask what we can do with love. I argue that the particular relationship that has been fashioned between population and healthcare system can be taken seriously as an asset for collective reimaginings of a sustainable welfare state for everyone, in which the broader societal supports for population health are understood as the investments they are. While brief details are given in each chapter of the underlying research methods, a methodological appendix offers a fuller account of each project, and additionally reflects on my own positionality as a lifelong 'participant observer' of the NHS.

2

Public opinion and the NHS

On 29 August 2022, *The Times* published a story headlined 'Britain falls out of love with the NHS: poll reveals three in five now expect delays' (Lintern and Wheeler, 2022). The report was of a YouGov poll commissioned by the newspaper to explore public attitudes to the NHS. Notably, none of the reported questions asked about, or even addressed, love at all. Online discussion of this article among commentators leapt from statements of declining satisfaction to the end of the NHS, and the inevitable importation of 'an American system of private medicine'; truly the spectre which haunts the feast of UK health policy debates (Lorne, 2022). Even responses which were more measured still quickly asserted that falling out of love might prompt people to 'opt out' and buy private care, undermining the service. A few months later, in November 2022, thinktank the King's Fund hosted a conference session of journalists and campaigners entitled 'Is the public falling out of love with the NHS?' and published a blog on the topic. Referring back to British Social Attitudes Survey data, the blog concluded 'the public's love for the NHS is being severely tested but it is far from being broken' (Wellings, 2022). Public support for the NHS is often evidenced in this way with reference to a fairly limited set of statistics. There remains a remarkable appetite for discussion and analysis of these data, promoted and contextualised by a handful of well-established health policy thinktanks.

This chapter explores the idea that these data constitute epistemic infrastructures (Bandola-Gill et al, 2022) which structure debates in the UK about public views of the NHS. The concept of epistemic infrastructure highlights how ways of knowing about, and of communicating knowledge on, any given issue can become embedded and entrenched in a context. Epistemic infrastructures are "the entities that make things known" (Bueger, 2015). I review quantitative analyses of public views on the NHS, but also seeks to contextualise these quantified reports of support, both in international comparison, and by investigating the organisations which fund and report such data in the UK. This role is particularly filled by three specialist health thinktanks: the Health Foundation, the King's Fund, and the Nuffield Trust. I explore the way in which questions often conflate 'satisfaction' and 'solidaristic' attitudes (Burlacu and Roescu, 2021) and argue that these data tend to close down conversations about the public and the NHS, rather than generate new insights. Drawing on research from scholars in sociology and in Science and Technology Studies (Osborne and

Rose, 1999; Law, 2009; Stone, 2020), I argue that these numbers are also performative. That is the act of measuring and reporting this information about public feelings, is not just descriptive, but purposeful, and has effects over and above a simple reporting of fact.

Public opinion and healthcare: the NHS in comparative perspective

Public opinion is understood as an important element of health system performance internationally (Reibling et al, 2019; Burlacu and Roescu, 2021), but also one that is particularly challenging to robustly quantify. Former KPMG Director Britnell's influential *In Search of the Perfect Health System* bemoans that in global rankings of performance:

> There is little attention paid to the recipients of health and healthcare – the patients and citizens. This is a serious omission and it is, unfortunately, the case that no universal patient satisfaction or experience scores exist for meaningful global comparisons. I hope this changes and countries collaborate more effectively in the future. (Britnell, 2015, p 2)

The potential of benchmarking (and potentially learning from success) in this area is complicated. First, and in common with many other aspects of health system performance, outcomes emerge from many decisions, both inside and outside the healthcare system, very few of which will be influenced by a desire to aid international comparison (Freeman, 2008; Schneider et al, 2021). Differences between the NHS in England, Northern Ireland, Scotland and Wales are a good example of how difficult comparison becomes when there is no political incentive to enable it by collecting consistent data (Bevan et al, 2014). There are also aspects of patient and citizen views that are particularly difficult to compare, based on their inherent subjectivity, and differences in what those statuses imply in different systems. In the UK, as this book will demonstrate, the population often act as stakeholders in the healthcare system, more than as demanding customers, and this orientation might influence the way we answer questions about healthcare.

When large-scale international comparisons do attempt to measure public views, they tend to conclude that support for the NHS in the UK is higher than support for healthcare systems in many European countries. Especially in the 2000s, satisfaction with the NHS was consistently above the European average (Burlacu and Roescu, 2021). However, it is worth noting that these figures are not quite such an outlier as claims about public affection for the NHS might suggest. Papanicolas et al (2019) compare the UK with nine high income country comparators: Australia, Canada, Denmark, France, Germany, the Netherlands, Sweden, Switzerland and the US. In 2017, 44 per cent of adult respondents think 'the healthcare system works well' in the UK. While close to the average for all high income countries the study compared, this is well below France (54 per cent), Germany (60 per cent) and Switzerland (58 per cent). This reflects a significant fall in this measure between 2010 and 2017. 63 per cent would have agreed with this statement in 2010, at which point the British public would have been the *most* satisfied with how their health system works within this study (Papanicolas et al, 2019).

Some of this distinctiveness is likely a function of our health system type: national health service-type systems do tend to have higher levels of public support than, for example, social insurance systems. Gevers et al (2000) conclude that 'support for an all-encompassing health care system is especially high in countries with highly developed national health services', citing Denmark and Sweden as other examples. What is more striking is that the UK continues to have high levels of public support for a national health service-type system within a broader context of our welfare state. The UK's relatively ungenerous income maintenance policies tend to place it as a 'liberal welfare regime', in which we might expect state provision to be minimal. And yet in the UK the NHS remains a highly state-centric model of healthcare, largely funded through general taxation.

Bambra has explained this as part of what she describes as a 'healthcare discrepancy' within scholarship on public attitudes to the welfare state (Bambra, 2005b) in which patterns of attitudes towards healthcare may be distinct from those towards other public provision. The classical welfare state typologies, starting with Esping-Anderson's (2013) 'worlds of welfare', have, Bambra argues, overstated the salience of cash transfers (also known as welfare payments or social security) and neglected the role of service-based provision (including healthcare, education and social care) (Bambra, 2005a; Jensen, 2008). Esping-Anderson's work takes as its starting point 'income maintenance' programmes but generalises from it to all social policy provision, without considering how the experience of service-based provision such as healthcare might shape attitudes towards it. Other examples of this discrepancy identified by Bambra (2005b) are Canada, New Zealand and to a lesser extent, Ireland. The discrepancy is often attributed to the way in which healthcare muddles straightforward notions of redistribution: public attitudes to spending on healthcare might be more positive because 'in the field of healthcare ... redistribution takes place primarily between risk groups, not between social classes' (Wendt et al, 2010, p 189).

Recently, scholars have also sought to be more specific about what kind of public attitudes are being measured. Reviewing literature on public opinion on healthcare in Europe, Burlacu and Roescu (2021) have proposed that academic research on public opinion and health systems consist of three 'disarticulated' literatures. These, they argue, have separately explored three different phenomena. The first is *solidarity*, which they describe as generalised normative feelings about the health system. A classic question to measure solidarity is one from the European Social Survey: in 2008 respondents were asked on a 10 point scale how far they think it is the government's responsibility to ensure adequate healthcare for the population. On this measure, the UK population was in the middle range across Europe, with highest support in Latvia and Lithuania, and the lowest in Switzerland. The second is *satisfaction*, which captures specific views on how well one's own or one's family's needs have been met by services within the health system. A classic question for this phenomenon would be the European Social Survey question 'please say what you think about the overall state of health services in this country nowadays?'. On this measure, the UK was towards the top of the distribution of European countries until 2012, with a significant drop in 2014 and 2016. The third is *salience*, which refers to how highly the health system features within one's own political priorities. That is, if a member of the public was asked to rank different areas of public policy as priorities for spending or attention, how would healthcare fare alongside education, defence, criminal justice or social security? The Eurobarometer survey asks people to select the two most important problems facing their country. In 2006, 41.6 per cent of UK respondents selected health. Thereafter this fell until 2012, when (in line with reducing satisfaction as outlined), it began gaining in political salience again.

While closely related, each of these facets of public opinion about health systems is interesting to different audiences. Salience, that is, how *much* people care about the NHS tells political actors not what substantive policies they should progress in order to get their party elected, but simply how much they need to be seen as 'pro-NHS'. And yet even satisfaction is a more complex phenomenon than it is often credited with being. As Wendt et al argue: 'The perceived (subjective) security to receive adequate medical treatment when in need can be considered to be highly relevant for the evaluation of the healthcare system in general' (2010). Thus satisfaction might not simply be a consumeristic evaluation of a single care experience, but rather a broader, retrospective *and* prospective sense of health security: 'Positive experiences with existing arrangements will lead to a favourable evaluation and can, in the long run, be expected to enhance trust not only in individuals (for example, certain healthcare providers) but in the overall institution' (Wendt et al, 2010). A lack of attention to the multi-faceted nature of public opinion on healthcare thus explains how news headlines can simultaneously report Britain 'falling out of love' with the NHS alongside robust support for its founding principles.

National research on public attitudes to the NHS

While international comparisons of public attitudes to healthcare fascinate health policy analysts, much discussion in the public realm focuses solely on data from within the UK. Quantified national accounts of public attitudes to the NHS come from a range of sources including the British Social Attitudes Survey, one-off opinion polling commissioned by thinktanks and newspapers, official NHS patient surveys, and occasional ad hoc projects by thinktanks. These are very different data sources.

One strand of knowledge about population perspectives on the NHS is contained within official NHS patient surveys. These have come and gone over the years and vary in their coverage across the UK (Care Quality Commission, 2022). Additionally they are focused, especially in secondary care settings, on recent patient experience rather than a more general sense of public views. One interesting exception to this, the 'Friends and Family Test', asks patients 'How likely are you to recommend our service to friends and family if they needed similar care or treatment?'. NHS organisations in England have been compelled to collect this data since 2014, despite consistent claims that it imposes a burden on providers without proving very useful (Robert et al, 2018). For the purposes of this chapter, the greater issue is that the Friends and Family Test remains focused on an assessment of a specific recent episode of care within one provider organisation, rather than broader attitudes to the NHS as a healthcare system.

By contrast, the British Social Attitudes Survey and one-off polls include questions on broader perspectives about the NHS as a healthcare system. The British Social Attitudes Survey is a large, annual survey that has run since 1983 (NatCen Social Research, 2022). It is managed by NatCen, a charitable social research organisation. A random probability survey, usually administered with in person interviews not online, the long-term nature of the survey enables it to track attitudes over time with a degree of robustness few other surveys can offer. Significantly, this survey operates across England, Wales and Scotland, excluding Northern Ireland but not, as with most commissioned polls, focusing only on England. Commissioned projects from commercial polling organisations (primarily Ipsos MORI) make up the rest of the data source of thinktank coverage of Britain's views of the NHS. These are very rarely random probability surveys, instead relying on demographically representative samples drawn from 'opt-in' panels of survey respondents (Curtice, 2016). In this section, I will review recent evidence from these different data sources and will also consider the single example identified of these thinktanks using qualitative methods to explore public views of the NHS.

British Social Attitudes Survey

The key question asked in the BSAS, which has been part of the survey since 1983, explores levels of satisfaction with the NHS. The question reads 'All in all, how satisfied or dissatisfied would you say you are with the way in which the National Health Service runs nowadays?'.

As shown in Figure 2.1, in the most recent report, this measure of satisfaction dropped off 17 percentage points between 2020 and 2021, from 53 per cent very or quite satisfied, to 36 per cent very or quite satisfied. This is, the report underlines, a dramatic finding: 'This fall in satisfaction is exceptional. It is the largest year-on-year fall in satisfaction since the question was first asked in 1983' (Wellings et al, 2022).

Since 2015 (although not every year), the survey has also sought to explore reasons for these stated levels of satisfaction. Respondents are given a different question depending on their stated level of satisfaction with the NHS. Respondents who are 'quite' or 'very' satisfied can choose up to three from a list of options. In the 2021 survey, the list is as shown in Figure 2.2.

The report notes that the top three reasons have been consistent since 2015, but with some statistically significant reordering between 2019 and 2021, with the NHS being 'free at the point of use' became a more popular reason, while satisfaction with waiting time was less often selected. The question for people who have stated that they are 'very' or 'quite' dissatisfied (see Figure 2.3) offers a slightly different list of potential reasons for respondents to select three from: for example there is no equivalent answer about the extent to which services are free or paid for at the point of use.

Again the report highlights that the top three reasons have remained unchanged in surveys since 2016, but highlights a change in order, with waiting times for appointments increasing to 'top' the list in 2021. The third most popular reason given – dissatisfaction because the government doesn't spend enough money on the NHS – is particularly intriguing, as it rejects the straightforward evaluation of a consumer (my NHS healthcare was not good enough) in favour of signalling political displeasure (my NHS healthcare was not good enough because the government has not funded it properly). The BSAS data thus suggests a significant decline in satisfaction with the NHS in recent years, and the reasons that people give for their verdict emphasise system features (cost and funding) alongside assessments of specific care received.

It is important to note that reports of BSAS data by the King's Fund and Nuffield Trust pay careful attention to claims, and make attempts to disaggregate views by population group. The reporting of the data is, at least below headline level, consistently robust and clear. For example, in 2020 the BSAS changed its standard questions in response to the pandemic, and conducted its survey online instead of face-to-face. The Nuffield Trust's reporting of this change is exemplary: a boxed section explains the changes in detail:

> The change in method brings a risk that differences in attitudes between the BSA in 2020 and 2021 and earlier years may be a consequence of the change of methodology. However, the 2021 data has been carefully

Figure 2.1: Public satisfaction with the NHS 1983–2021

Question asked: 'All in all, how satisfied or dissatisfied would you say you are with the way in which the National Health Service runs nowadays?'

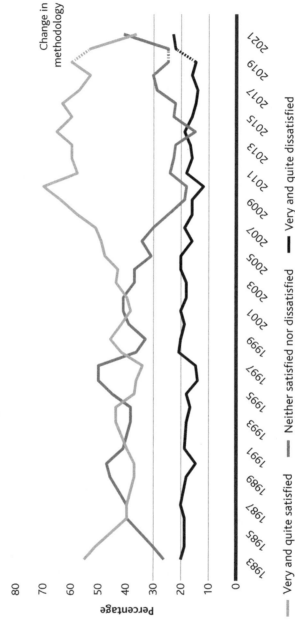

— Very and quite satisfied   — Neither satisfied nor dissatisfied   — Very and quite dissatisfied

Source: The King's Fund and Nuffield Trust analysis of NatCen Social Research's BSA survey data. 2021 sample size 3,112. This question was not asked in 1985, 1988 and 1992; 'Don't know' and Refusal' responses are not shown; in 2021 these response categories were selected by 0.5 per cent of respondents. Data has been carefully weighted to minimise differences due to the change in methodology between 2020 and previous years.

Figure 2.2: Reasons for satisfaction with the NHS overall in 2021

Question asked: 'You said you are satisfied with the way in which the National Health Service runs nowadays. Why do you say that? You can choose up to three options.'

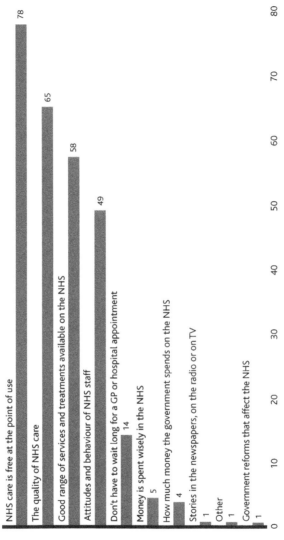

Percentage of respondents stating that they were 'very' or 'quite' satisfied

Source: The King's Fund and Nuffield Trust analysis of NatCen Social Research's BSA survey data. Sample size = 410. This question was asked to respondents who said they were 'quite' or 'very' satisfied with the way the NHS runs nowadays within the random third of the overall sample selected to answer the health and social care module of questions.

Figure 2.3: Reasons for dissatisfaction with the NHS overall in 2021

Question asked: 'You said you are dissatisfied with the way in which the National Health Service runs nowadays. Why do you say that? You can choose up to three options.'

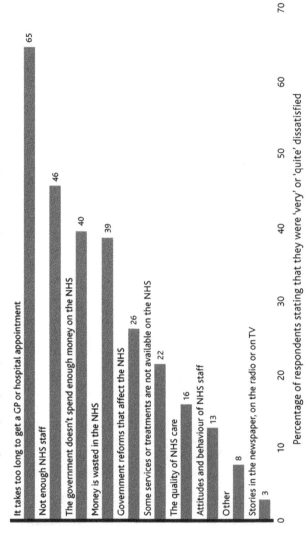

Percentage of respondents stating that they were 'very' or 'quite' dissatisfied

Source: The King's Fund and Nuffield Trust analysis of NatCen Social Research's BSA survey data. Sample size = 400. This question was asked to respondents who said they were 'quite' or 'very' dissatisfied with the way the NHS runs nowadays within the random third of the overall sample selected to answer the health and social care module of questions.

weighted to ensure this risk has been minimised. The methodology section explains further reasons to be confident in making comparisons between years. (Wellings et al, 2022, p 4)

This rather dry technical content, flagging the need for caution in interpreting results, is featured in both the prologue to the webpage and the first sentence of the substantive content.

The academic orientation of the BSAS does stand out when comparing with the broader corpus of reports on public views of the NHS on thinktank websites. While most of the reporting relies on descriptive statistics, British Social Attitudes Survey reports are the only ones which routinely describe statistical significance and transparently discuss the significant limitations of the sample size (in 2021, the NHS questions were answered by 3,112 people). For example, for ethnic groups, the report differentiates satisfaction between people identifying as 'mixed/other' (33 per cent very or quite satisfied), 'white' (36 per cent), 'Asian' (37 per cent) and 'Black' (36 per cent). The report explains 'these are the most granular levels of ethnicity captured in the survey'. Due to the small numbers of ethnic minority respondents in the survey (there were 63 Black respondents in 2021), it isn't possible to ascertain whether changes in satisfaction between survey are statistically significant for any group except those identifying as white (Wellings et al, 2022, p 9). The BSAS sample size is, as we will see, larger than those routinely used for commissioned polls, as well as more robustly recruited. However its ongoing weakness in exploring ethnic minority perspectives seems increasingly problematic given improved evidence of racism in healthcare (Kar, 2020; Black Equity Organisation and Clearview Research, 2022). People with disabilities are not disaggregated in the report at all. While reports do make some effort to disaggregate the data by age, gender and party political affiliation, the headline reporting, and certainly content that makes it out of the published report and into media coverage, remains focused on a singular public and simple descriptive statistics.

Commissioned polls

Beyond reporting the BSAS data, thinktanks and other organisations also commission and conduct additional research on public opinion on the NHS on an ad hoc basis. Rather than the academic standards of the BSAS, polling reports generally state adherence to the Market Research Society standards, designed for political polling (Mortimore and Wells, 2017). Given the priority placed by all the thinktanks on English policy, both because of their London base and due to its much greater size within the UK, commissioned polls also tend to focus only on respondents in England. Reports are largely oriented to influencing Westminster decisions, and often timed to coincide with elections or changes of government (Ipsos MORI Public Affairs, 2019; Buzelli et al, 2022). Special polls were also commissioned to commemorate the 70th anniversary of the NHS in 2018: all three thinktanks teamed up with the Institute for Fiscal Studies to commission a poll to explore perceptions of the NHS's future (The Health Foundation, 2018). In 2019 the Health Foundation repeated many of the questions in commissioned polling from Ipsos MORI, with a face-to-face survey of 2000 people (Ipsos MORI Public Affairs, 2019).

On balance, these reports supplement rather than challenge or offer new perspectives to the report based on the BSAS. The questions in commissioned polls are similar to the key BSAS question wording on satisfaction: 'All in all, how satisfied or dissatisfied would you say you are with the way in which the NHS runs nowadays'. In a series of commissioned polls, respondents are asked instead: 'I'd like you to think about your own experience and everything you have seen, heard or read recently. Do you think the general standard of care provided by the NHS over the last 12 months has been getting (scale from slightly better to much worse).' This question is more specifically focused on standard of care, while the BSAS question might reasonably prompt reflection on, for example, broader system issues such as accessibility or equity of care. The prompt to think beyond one's immediate experiences to 'everything you have seen, heard or read recently' is another difference, as well as an explicit focus on whether things are perceived to be getting better or worse. Comparing results with 2017 data, the 2019 report states that fewer respondents describe care having got worse, and additionally that 'when thinking about the future, the public are slightly less pessimistic than they were in 2017'. Although the key points listed in the report's executive summary focus only on headline findings for the whole sample of respondents, inside the report it is also noted that

> People who have used an NHS service in the last year and people with disabilities are particularly negative about the standard of services over the last year, which is concerning as they may actually have seen declines in standards rather than making assumptions about them (for example, based on media coverage). (Ipsos MORI Public Affairs, 2019, p 6)

Another recurring concern of commissioned polling questions goes beyond people's satisfaction with the current state of the NHS, and instead probes how respondents feel about its 'ideal' or 'founding principles'. The Health Foundation polling repeatedly investigates support for what they describe as 'the principles underpinning the NHS'. The question asks respondents, on a scale of 1–10, to express their agreement with the statement 'The government should support a national health system that is tax funded, free at the point of use, and providing comprehensive care for all citizens.'

Agreement with this statement has risen in the waves of this survey, from 60 per cent in 2015 up to 72 per cent in 2019 (Ipsos MORI Public Affairs, 2019). The report, implying that these principles were highly supported historically, suggests 'the public feel as strongly connected to the principles underpinning the NHS as ever'. In fact, within the 2017–19 period, the data actually show a notable increase in this measure.

Intriguingly in other Ipsos MORI polling (The Health Foundation and Ipsos, 2022b), this question is disaggregated by principle and the wording altered:

- The NHS should be free at the point of delivery (91 per cent support in 2017, 89 per cent in 2022);
- The NHS should provide a comprehensive service available to everyone (85 per cent support in 2017, 88 per cent in 2022);
- The NHS should be primarily funded through taxation (88 per cent support in 2017, 85 per cent in 2022).

These data are drawn from two different polls with different methods, and so no conclusions can be drawn from the comparative stability of these figures. Ipsos MORI polling for the King's Fund in 2017 asks respondents which of the following statements best reflects their thinking about the NHS: 77 per cent select 'the NHS is crucial to British society and we must do everything we can to maintain it' while 23 per cent select 'the NHS was a great project but we probably can't maintain it'. Setting to one side the crudeness of the question, the report's interpretation is 'The public is still bought into the ideal of the NHS and are keen to protect it.' The report suggests that this polling question goes back as far as 2000, including in a former Department of Health-funded 'perceptions of the NHS tracker', and the proportions are, as the report states, 'remarkably stable', with a low of 73 and a high of 79 per cent (Ipsos MORI for the King's Fund, 2017).

What is striking about these ad hoc additional polling projects are their strong similarities to the British Social Attitudes Survey questions, with reported findings mirroring the framing of the BSAS. Satisfaction ('is the NHS providing a good service?') remains the primary lens through which public perspectives are viewed. They generate findings which are similar enough to BSAS not to offer novel insights, and yet with wording that is different enough to make it difficult to draw conclusions over time. By including additional questions probing 'the founding principles' of the NHS – and consistently finding high levels of declared support for these – the polls do, though, shed some light on the solidaristic attitudes of the sample towards healthcare provision. Headline reporting of these polls also remains primarily interested in a headline figure which can represent a singular imagined public, and track its (singular, imagined) satisfaction over time. The executive summary of a tailored report on 'What the new

Government should know' (Buzelli et al, 2022) reports only four over-arching views attributed to 'the public', and makes no reference to how views might vary across the population. While reports of ad hoc polling in the 2010s demonstrate even less focus than the British Social Attitudes Survey reports in disaggregating responses across demographic groups, there is a noticeable shift in 2022. Reports from the Health Foundation's newest programme make claims about how attitudes vary by ethnicity and region, offering a new, and overdue, focus on diversity in attitudes (The Health Foundation and Ipsos, 2022b).

Occasionally, one-off projects pursue a different approach. One report on public expectations of healthcare shifts into using polling, curiously enough, to show how wrong the public are about the NHS (Duffy, 2021). A report from King's College London's Policy Institute and the Health Foundation reports a poll of 2,056 English adults conducted by Savanta ComRes at the height of the 2020 winter lockdown. The conclusion page is titled 'Perceptions vs reality: what the public get wrong about the state of the NHS and the health of the nation'. Reporting the data, it begins: 'People in England have an overwhelmingly positive view of the NHS. There is almost universal agreement (84 per cent) that the health service is one of the best in the world, and the public have a hugely favourable opinion of the care that they and their family have access to' (Duffy, 2021). The report acknowledges that this might have been skewed by the pandemic context, because views of service quality were less positive before the pandemic. It then goes on to identify negative 'misperceptions' ('the average guess is that 52 per cent of people wait at least 18 weeks for hospital treatment, when the reality is 17%') and positive 'misperceptions' ('The public believe that life expectancy in the UK compares more favourably to other OECD nations than it does in reality'). It isn't clear from this report what significance is being attributed to the public's 'misperceptions', but it is reminiscent of longstanding arguments that public 'deficits' of knowledge justify either educating, or ignoring, their views entirely (Wynne, 2006; Kerr et al, 2007).

Searching the thinktank websites identified only one example of qualitative methods being employed to explore public views on the NHS. The King's Fund, again working with Ipsos MORI, conducted what they variously describe as 'deliberative workshops' or 'discussion events' in England in 2018 (Ewbank et al, 2018). These were attended by 75 people recruited to include a range of self-reported use of the NHS, levels of satisfaction, status as a carer and political affiliations. These events focused on perceptions of the NHS in general, of expectations of the NHS, and (somewhat peculiarly, given the extensive evidence that health outcomes are primarily determined neither by healthcare nor individual behaviour (Marmot, 2010)) of the balance of responsibility between governments and individuals for personal health.

While brief and basic, the report still gives a sense of the richness and complexity which could be brought to these conversations when public views are explored on their own terms, rather than measured against pre-existing yardsticks. The section of the report which considers views on the NHS in general, and 'its role in Britain today' describes pride in the NHS as 'part of our heritage', as a 'safety net' and as a 'fundamental right'. Participants also, though, describe the service as being 'under pressure': 'Despite feeling grateful for and positive about the NHS, some people were more negative about their day-to-day experiences with the service' (Ewbank et al, 2018). More negative views emphasised waiting times, and concerns about efficiency. In common with polls, the events also explored founding principles, which were summarised as 'a comprehensive service available to all, free at the point of delivery, and primarily funded through taxation'. These were felt by participants to still be correct, but with some discussion about whether they remain achievable in a changing population (the report specifies participants referencing increasing life expectancy and a perceived increase in immigration as pertinent here). This is in agreement with polling in which 77 per cent of respondents stated 'the NHS is crucial to British society and we must do everything we can to maintain it' (King's Fund, 2017).

Perhaps most interesting, participants were asked to work in age-segregated groups to come up with 'new deals' for the NHS and the public, in which they put forward a broad range of proposals including suggesting that the NHS should look for additional sources of funding beyond taxation. No detail is offered in the report for whether limits were placed on the additional sources of funding, or indeed whether this is understood as a threat to the progressive taxation–funded basis of current funding (Ruane, 1997). Despite these intriguing possibilities for a more complex discussion on how publics feel about the NHS, the reporting is, as so often in this genre of policy-relevant output, brief and only lightly contextualised. Insights about public debate about the future of the NHS remain overwhelmingly stuck in a binary dead end: in, or out, of love.

Polling data as epistemic infrastructure

This analysis demonstrates both the sheer quantity of these assessments of how Britain feels about the NHS and the relatively narrow parameters through which that relationship is viewed. The overwhelming focus is on satisfaction, with more solidaristic questions channelled through the particular lens of the 'founding principles'. The bifurcation suggests either confusion, or a lack of interest, in how answers to the questions 'are you happy with the care you receive from NHS services' and 'do you support the NHS as a public service' are related (Wendt et al, 2010). The inclusion in the British Social Attitudes Survey of whether media stories are a reason for (dis)satisfaction

(Wellings et al, 2022) exemplifies this muddle. People don't tend to agree that media coverage is one of the top three influences on their feelings about the NHS, but of course media coverage is inexplicably entangled with *how* we know the NHS. Fortunate people who go months, even years, without personally experiencing the NHS, might not be personally aware of things like growing waiting times. However, the chances of someone in the UK never *hearing* anyone talking about these issues seems close to none. We encounter the NHS discursively as well as by using services, and for swathes of the population, our knowledge of it is shaped as much by societal discussions as by visits to a hospital.

One way to contextualise quantitative measurement of public attitudes to the NHS is to employ the idea that these data comprise an 'epistemic infrastructure' of knowledge about the public and the NHS. Put simply, these surveys and reports structure the ways in which the relationship between healthcare system and population is understood. Utilising the concept to reflect on the Sustainable Development Goals in global governance, Bandola-Gill et al (2022) propose that an epistemic infrastructure consists both of the practical aspects of how knowledge is generated (what they call the 'materialities of measurement') and the broader context of people and organisations around the data (the 'interlinkages'). This approach brings the broader context of this data into view: the 'materialities of measurement' consisting of the financing and the practical design and delivery of polls and surveys; the interlinkages between journalists, thinktanks and broader policy communities that fund, commission, report and generate debate about the data. While the concept of epistemic infrastructures has been most often used to trace the international journeys of expert knowledge (Bueger, 2015; Tichenor et al, 2022), it also has significant potential to enhance our understanding at the national level. The advantage of this approach is that it understands the knowledge generated through these activities holistically, embedded into both the way it is generated and the way these data act in the world (as 'knowledge products'). This section explores each in turn.

The materialities of these measurements – that is, how this approach is built into the construction of a public view of the NHS through particular research methods and questions – revolves centrally around the UK's health policy thinktanks: the Nuffield Trust, the King's Fund, and the Health Foundation. Together, they have an established body of work on public opinion and the NHS over several decades. Each year, they provide extensive analysis of the publication of the British Social Attitudes Survey questions on the NHS, speculating about what in the broader policy landscape might have caused a rise or fall in satisfaction. Their role goes beyond reporting these data: in 2011, the Department of Health declined to continue funding the module of the British Social Attitudes Survey on views on the NHS, and the King's Fund stepped in to do so (Young, 2011). It was later joined by the Nuffield

Trust, and in 2022 the two thinktanks continued to share funding of the question module. These efforts allow the continuation of the key question asked since 1983 – 'all in all, how satisfied or dissatisfied would you say you are with the way in which the National Health Service runs nowadays?' – and the possibility of adding additional questions. In 2021 they added questions about priorities for the NHS and 'the extent to which they think the founding principles of the NHS should still apply' (Wellings et al, 2022). Enabling a consistent question to be asked across decades generates remarkable data, as described earlier in this chapter. However this, and the preoccupation with framing broader discussions about the NHS in terms of 'founding principles', also structures and limits what can be known through this survey.

As described, the Health Foundation's approach instead has mostly involved commissioning its own polling from Ipsos MORI. This included polling for the 2015, 2017 and 2019 General Elections, and for the NHS's 70th anniversary in 2018: they 'wanted to conduct further public perceptions research to add to its "library"' (The Health Foundation, 2018). This research included updating some trend data from previous years, as well as collecting new data on emerging issues. In the wake of the COVID-19 pandemic, the Health Foundation launched a new two-year programme of 'public perceptions research' again in partnership with Ipsos MORI. Stating that the pandemic has prompted 'major shifts in public attitudes towards health, the NHS and social care', this programme asks: 'But how might public attitudes continue to change? And what might this mean for policy makers working to plot a course out of the pandemic, learn from the response so far and repair the social and economic damage caused by the virus?' (The Health Foundation, 2022). This programme brings together multiple polls into what is termed an Expectations Tracker, depicting trends over time. However, as the report states: 'Please note that methodologies differ and so comparisons are indicative rather than direct'' (The Health Foundation and Ipsos, 2022b, p 2).

Starting with the most basic level of the materialities of these measurements, the choice of questions asked shapes answers given in a survey. Surveys are expensive undertakings and inevitably directed towards what are perceived to be the most salient issues by those running and funding them (Henderson and Jones, 2021). This is unavoidable: there is no neutral question wording that can tap into our innermost consciousness and extract a quantifiable response like a nurse might a blood sample. High quality surveys are transparent about this, but, especially in commercial polling, question wording is much less transparent. This explains why prominent academics are often critical of commercial opinion polling, especially when results are reported without context in front page news (Jennings and Wlezien, 2018). In the UK we are fortunate to have the long-running and robust British Social Attitudes Survey to rely upon, which, as described, has some consistent question wording over time. We are additionally fortunate to have thinktanks who transparently report their own role in funding particular questions and who clearly explain when results over time are not directly comparable, because a question has changed. However, answers to survey questions, like all research questions, remain artefacts of measurement, not natural phenomena.

The consistent interest in, and time and money provided for, measuring public attitudes to the NHS gives thinktanks a key role in structuring the debate about those attitudes. This makes understanding the role of thinktanks within UK health policy debates a crucial part of the jigsaw of understanding how Britain loves the NHS. The three main thinktanks, the King's Fund, the Health Foundation and the Nuffield Trust, are funded by varying sizes of charitable endowments, and supplement this with 'soft money' consultancy and grant income (Shaw et al, 2015). This means that the more solidly endowed thinktanks sometimes commission and fund work from the more precarious ones, and that they sometimes work in partnership. As well as these variations within their roles, their strategic foci shift over time with changes in leadership and context: these organisations are not static actors within the health policy landscape.

A handful of thoughtful studies have explored UK's health policy thinktanks' peculiar knowledge positions. A focus on research and analysis tasks allows health thinktanks to present their outputs (for example reports, events, press releases) as what Shaw et al describe as 'a view from nowhere' (Shaw et al, 2015). The conclusions that they draw are presented as being neutral, when in practice these organisations are enmeshed within complex relationships of dependency with opinion formers and decision-makers (Maybin, 2016). In these, the issues which become deemed as 'matters of concern' are iteratively formed: thinktanks may put some issues onto the policy agenda, but they also learn what is already appearing on the agenda and shift their considerable powers of analysis towards those issues in search of influence. These are not malign processes, although they are worthy of scrutiny and transparency (Shaw et al, 2014). Financial independence is not the only marker of neutrality, and thinktanks trade in influence (Stone, 1996). To do this, they must balance 'keeping distance' and 'arranging proximity' to power (Jezierska and Sörbom, 2021).

In the context of these reflections about the shifting substantive and organisational priorities of UK health thinktanks, it is striking that public opinion on the NHS is such a consistent interest across the Health Foundation, the Nuffield Trust and the King's Fund over the years. Responding to sustained media and political interest in reporting and debating the topic, these organisations play significant roles in making public opinion on the NHS known. A search of the organisational websites in October 2021 found a significant track record of reports, events, blogs and briefings on the topic, from all three. The language used to describe these reports varies. While all three discuss public attitudes (presumably due to the foundational role of the BSAS within this epistemic infrastructure): the Nuffield Trust additionally employs public satisfaction, perspectives, thinking and acceptance; the King's Fund discusses views, opinion and satisfaction; and most expansively, the Health Foundation variously explores mood, perceptions, expectations, thinking, views and support. The choice of language might not be consciously strategic, but the consequences are significant. Osborne and Rose (1999) note the emergence of the idea that what most needed to be measured was 'opinion', denoting something considered and informed, and they distinguish it from closely related alternatives like 'attitudes'. Attitudes, they argue, denote more reflex, deeply held (and even in some cases concealed) perspectives. They identify the way in which quantified representations of 'mass opinion' became integral to political and economic functioning, as both politicians and businesses look to understand and act upon them.

Once these data are generated, the nexus of health policy thinktanks and related commentators form an epistemic community (Bandola-Gill et al, 2022) in which the meaning and significance of the results is generated and debated. Scholars have argued that the very idea of public opinion is a phenomenon significantly generated by the industries of market research during the 20th century. For Osborne and Rose, the industry which sprang up around public opinion generated an illusory image of solidity:

> Opinion here hardly referred to anything beyond itself; it became, so to speak, something that was thing-like in itself, something that existed in its own right and, with the right technical resources and procedural methods, could be known and measured. In other words, opinion was something that simply emerged as a fact in its own right from the collectivity of people's individual opinions. (Osborne and Rose, 1999, p 387)

To help trace what they call 'the creation of public opinion', they point to other possibilities, or roads not taken, in this emergent science of quantifying what people think. They unpick the standardisation of the innovation of sampling theory in the 1940s, and the increasing acceptance of the notion that this, well-constructed, could stand in for how a whole population feels. John Law makes similar arguments about this, describing it as a 'romantic notion' in which society as a collectivity is 'a more or less coherent whole that both contains and is emergent from the interactions between the individual elements that make it up' (Law, 2009). This romanticism, he argues 'assumes that this larger context can be known in a manner that is single, centred, explicit, homogenous, and abstract' (Law, 2009).

Beyond the creation of an industry of public opinion, Osborne and Rose argue that one of the most significant effects of the institutionalisation of public opinion has been on publics themselves. Opinion polling has, they assert, caused 'the creation of "opinioned" persons. … If humans themselves are changing, there is no obvious stable point to visualize a "before" and "after" scenario, no static dimension with a fixed scale allowing the measurement of relative success or failure. We are all "opinioned" now' (Osborne and Rose, 1999). By this account, the idea that, as members of the UK population, we should hold opinions on the NHS becomes a self-fulfilling prophecy. Furthermore, the structures which run surveys and report this data encourage a particular way of thinking about how we might value the NHS, focusing on our (personal) satisfaction with a service and squeezing space for broader debates about how we might value healthcare now and in the future. This is an artefact of an industry that has collected that opinion, in particular ways, and reported it widely.

Conclusion

Data on the public's opinion of the NHS serves as a seemingly endless catalyst for media discussion and political debate in the UK. UK politics is not alone in according quantitative evidence disproportionate weight within its policy debates; even quantitative specialists often express frustration at the way that a 'killer graph' or figure can take on a life of its own (Jerrim and de Vries, 2017). However, this chapter has demonstrated that in the UK our debates about how the public values the NHS have been heavily shaped by a relatively limited set of statistics, promoted and contextualised by a handful of thinktanks then further amplified by media coverage. In weighing and measuring stated attitudes to the NHS, surveys lump together more differentiated experiences into a question of degrees of 'satisfaction'. The potential for exploring more solidaristic rationales for feelings about the NHS is transposed instead into a debate about adherence to 'founding principles', which risks confusing nostalgic and optimistic responses. Furthermore, despite improved efforts to disaggregate perspectives across different population groups, the wider reporting of these data consistently reverts to a series of statements about a singular public view. That such reports are usually based on robust statistics from a well-respected social survey does not mean that they are the final word, or an unarguable truth, when it comes to how the British public feels about the NHS.

Conceptualising these data as epistemic infrastructures asserts that they do not only let us know how the public feels, but structure the possibility for how public views might be known. The data has value, but its dominance in debates about the NHS is limiting. The very commitment to the dataset's quantitative rigour, and to its comparisons to last year's data, last government's data, data from the periods of largesse or austerity, prevents our grasp of this social phenomenon shifting and improving. The 'seductions of quantification' (Merry, 2016) are often described in relation to international comparisons: a field in which health system comparisons are an enduringly fascinating topic (Freeman, 2008; Vindrola-Padros and Whiteford, 2021). However in the case of public opinion data on the NHS, it is the potential for comparisons over time that seems to fascinate and absorb media coverage. Newspapers ponder us falling in and out of love with the NHS with similar focus to the love affairs of minor celebrities, but correlated instead with policy, with spending and with performance measures. The numerical tracking of opinion creates an illusion of 'order, mobility, stability, combinability and precision. Numbers transform complex issues into readily auditable objects' (Bandola-Gill et al, 2022). And yet, as this chapter has demonstrated, we cannot escape the instability and incommensurability of language in this area: embedded as it is in question wording, our own articulation of phenomena as 'opinioned people' (Osborne and Rose, 1999), and in the epistemic communities that report and debate the phenomenon.

This epistemic infrastructure is more than the 'attitudinal context' for policy decisions (Cooper and Burchardt, 2022). They have political value in helping organisations justify or oppose reforms: informing politicians that they must be seen to preserve healthcare spending even as the services that prevent ill-health are crumbling around the NHS. Sometimes, by emphasising the ways in which public respondents' expressed attitudes are at odds with evidence, they help organisations make a case for paying *less* attention to public preferences. However this epistemic infrastructure also shapes publics. With reference to the example of Canada, Marmor et al (2010) refute the idea that health systems exist as reflections of foundational societal values: 'Social and political institutions, once created, develop lives of their own.' There is as Burlacu and Roescu (2021) note, a 'two-way relationship between public opinion and health policies'. By exploring the work these polls do in their broader socio-political context, this chapter is also about how we come to know, as a society, our feelings about the NHS. Reflecting on the associated but distinct phenomenon of how a 'patient' perspective on any given issue might emerge, Pols (2005) stresses that any particular articulation is 'not something that is "already there" in the mind of the patient, to be put into words … the patient perspective (or any other perspective) can be seen as being produced in a practical situation marked by specific possibilities and constraints'. She describes the way in which expressing an opinion can be performative, and not merely a linear communication of a pre-existing fact. Pols offers the example, also very familiar in Britain, of expressing an opinion about the weather, in a fashion that is so banal as to be almost nonsensical as communication, but highly functional as a 'binding' device. I think we can understand that stating and debating our views about the NHS has similar functions, generating a (sometimes illusory) sense of shared experience and values, as much as shedding light on the issue of how we feel about whatever we might mean by 'the NHS'.

The rest of this book explores other possibilities for thinking about public relationships with the NHS more expansively, and in a fashion that better connects up the parts of human experience. This rejects a quest to better pin down and analyse public views from within the 'all-embracing episteme' (Law, 2009), of 'thingified' public opinion. My approach prioritises understanding politics as what Latour (2005) calls 'matters of concern' rather than 'matters of fact'. For Freeman and de Voß (2015), 'social ordering is now achieved by seeking to establish valid representations of reality and shared acceptance of the factual conditions of collective action, rather than political representations of a collective will'. This book pursues an alternative, and more ambitious approach. Alongside or as well as trying to refine methods of surveying public opinion on the NHS, we can acknowledge the role these data play within entrenched institutional narratives (Tuohy, 2023) of our healthcare system. Doing so might create space for other routes to understand and act on public love for the NHS.

3

Fundraising for the NHS

In Chapter 2, I explored the public opinion data which shapes our understanding of public sentiments around the NHS. This chapter turns to the first of the four sets of practices through which this book seeks to explore Britain's love for the NHS: the donation and fundraising of money to gift to the NHS. The UK NHS is enmeshed in complex relations with the voluntary and community sector, who may act as service providers, funders of innovation and research and, sometimes, funders of particular forms of provision (Mohan and Gorsky, 2001; Powell, 2007). My focus in this chapter is more modest and specific. I focus on processes through which members of the public in the UK donate or fundraise money for NHS organisations. This practice has a number of peculiarities: it can be understood as a form of self-taxation, in that one cannot in the UK donate to the NHS in order to receive preferential services beyond those available to the whole population served. This distinguishes it from informal payments within the health system (Cohen et al, 2022).

The practices of NHS fundraising do, though, bear some resemblance to individual healthcare crowdfunding for care that is not (yet) mainstream provision (Barcelos, 2020; Kerr et al, 2021). In this mode, fundraising platforms can be interpreted as stages on which illness narratives are performed, and combined within narratives of the individual's good character and worthiness (Paulus and Roberts, 2018; Kenworthy, 2021). Discursive strategies to promote the deservingness of a cause (Kerr et al, 2021) can create a burden on the already sick individual, who may feel that through carrying out a campaign they are opened up to scrutiny to prove their legitimacy and their gratitude to donors (Kenworthy, 2021; Kerr et al, 2021). There is also evidence that the financial success of individual crowdfunders is strongly related to how wealthy a community the fundraiser lives in: that is, that crowdfunding exacerbates inequalities in health (Igra et al, 2021). While much sociological literature is highly critical of crowdfunding for healthcare, it is also acknowledged to be generative of 'new solidarities' between people who share a particular medical condition (Kerr et al, 2021). Some scholars have gone further, identifying the positive social support that crowdfunding can generate for fundraisers, alongside a potentially 'empowering' identity shift as fundraisers share their vulnerabilities to increase awareness of their conditions (Gonzales et al, 2018).

Another resonance is between the donations analysed in this chapter and what in the USA has been described as 'grateful patient' (Jagsi et al, 2020) fundraising by hospitals. In the US, healthcare philanthropy is a significant phenomenon, due, of course, in no small part to the absence of universal healthcare (Schneider et al, 2008). Data collected annually by the Healthcare Philanthropy Association is expensively paywalled, but peer-reviewed research reports that in 2016, American health care institutions received $10.1 billion in charitable gifts (Collins et al, 2018). Grounded in the overall *lack* of public funding within the US healthcare system, hospital leaders are urged to build a 'culture of philanthropy' within their organisations which incorporates annual giving (through fundraising events, for example), major giving, including from businesses, and estate giving, including legacies (McGinly, 2008). This 'system-wide culture' is described as requiring every member of staff in a healthcare institution, not only recognising that philanthropy is critical for the organisation, but actively playing a role in the process of fundraising. Clinicians are at the centre of this: 'They must be willing to work with development staff to cultivate donors while protecting the physician-patient relationship' (Hook and Mapp, 2005). This has led to debates about, and some tentative recommendations to solve, the ethical risks of doctor-patient conversations about philanthropy (Collins et al, 2018; Jagsi, 2019). A recent survey suggested that public attitudes to these practices were less permissive than the current legal framework: '83.2% strongly agreed or agreed that physicians talking with their patients about donating may interfere with the patient-physician relationship' (Jagsi et al, 2020).

These examples highlight some of the intrinsic tensions involved in charitable fundraising for healthcare. While charitable fundraising is a longstanding feature of the NHS it has become increasingly visible, and significantly 'nationalised' in focus, since 2018, with a substantial intensification of activity since the COVID-19 pandemic. The motivating question for this chapter, then, is: how might we understand these contemporary practices of donating money or fundraising for the NHS as an act of love? I begin by reviewing the complicated history of voluntary funds within the NHS. Then, I share an analysis of crowdfunding pages created by members of the public to raise money for the NHS in the early months of the COVID-19 pandemic, before concluding by reflecting on what kind of love, and what constructed imaginary of the NHS, is revealed within NHS fundraising.

The past and present of NHS fundraising

The COVID-19 pandemic greatly raised the profile of charitable fundraising for the NHS. However, NHS charities, known by other names, have existed since the creation of the NHS, and indeed many evolved from voluntary associations which predated it (Gorsky et al, 2005; Gorsky and Sheard, 2006). They began as endowments, large financial balances held by voluntary hospitals which predated the NHS. Gosling (2017) has demonstrated the complex interrelations of payment by patients and philanthropic funding in the decades immediately preceding the creation of the NHS. Fundraising events such as Hospital Saturday or Hospital Sunday, often with an explicitly religious bent, were widespread across the UK (Cherry, 2000; Piggott, 2022). In the negotiations around the formation of the NHS, newly formed NHS organisations were allowed to retain inherited charitable balances to enhance or supplement statutory NHS services. The continuation of these charitable endeavours within the NHS has been an recurrent source of controversy since the earliest debates about a tax-funded health service (Mohan, 2002; Webster, 2002). Like so much of the NHS, the retained endowments were a solution to competing interests, with well-funded former voluntary hospitals, especially in London, keen to keep and use their pre-NHS endowments, despite the aspirations of centralised planning (Prochaska, 1997). In the 1980s, the Conservative government liberalised the rules against active fundraising (Lattimer, 1996) and there followed significant and rapid growth of a handful of the richest endowments into some of the most recognisable charity brands in the UK, most notably the Great Ormond Street Hospital Children's Charity.

This expansion was, however, deeply uneven across the country. In 2020, the average NHS Charity in London had total income and endowments of £8.7million, while for NHS charities in Yorkshire & Humber, the average was £869,000 (Carrington, 2021). A recent analysis on trust-level variation in England by Bowles et al (2023) explored variation by trusts of different size, location, and also sector. This identified strong inequalities around the 'sector' of organisation: that is, whether the NHS Trust was specialist, community, ambulance or mental health. This analysis demonstrated

> for most acute trusts, charitable income is equivalent to between 0.1% and 1% of total Trust income. Notably the level of charitable income tends to be much lower for ambulance, community and mental health Trusts. Indeed, for the majority of Trusts in these sectors, it is an order of magnitude lower than for the majority of acute trusts: charitable income represents only between 0.01% and 0.1% of total Trust income. In contrast, for the majority of specialist trusts, charitable income is considerably higher, representing between 1% and 10% of total income. (Bowles et al, 2013)

London NHS charities were found to have distinctively high charitable income, even when hospital size and sector are controlled for, suggesting a regional effect distinct from the presence of several very large NHS charities (Prochaska, 1997). Nonetheless, despite these differences in scale and emphasis, the 250 NHS charities across the UK fulfil broadly similar roles in the health system. They supplement statutory healthcare provision, often funding 'add ons' to patient care (such as arts in health) and staff development (such as training) (New Philanthropy Capital, 2019). Rather than being a creature of health policy, consciously designed with a goal of supplementing funding from general taxation, one can understand NHS charities as shaped by shifting regulation in the decades since the creation of the NHS (Möller and Abnett, under review).

Alongside these fundraising efforts from within the NHS, the landscape is further complicated by more conventionally voluntary associations known as Leagues of Friends, which have long raised money independently to support their local hospitals. Millward (2023) states that in 2013 there were around 1500 Leagues of Friends in the UK, and argues that the work of these eclectic organisations offers a lens on public roles that were neither consumeristic nor primarily activist in orientation. In a 2019 study, Paine et al (2019) identified that English community hospitals had a median voluntary income of £15,632 per year via their Leagues of Friends, but that overall charitable income for these organisations has been in decline since the mid-1990s. While small sums in comparison with overall hospital budgets, the persistence of these efforts to support local NHS institutions, often driven by a small group of committed, often elderly and middle-class, community members, is intriguing.

Fundraising work also has political consequences beyond the material facts of what this money can buy. Leagues of Friends are often adept at mobilising a broader section of the local population when hospitals are perceived as 'under threat' (Paine et al, 2019; Stewart, 2019). In one case study I conducted of a community hospital in Scotland, the local League of Friends were frank and straightforward in their assessment of the impact of their substantial local fundraising in 'saving' the hospital from a previous closure proposal:

> We were showing ourselves to be politically very effective and I've got no doubt that was a factor in the equation. We'd also shown ourselves generally as a community campaigning group to have a lot of support which is well evidenced, you know, with the number of collections there are at funerals, the number of people that turn up for our events, the number of legacies that are left to us. (Male campaigner, quoted in Stewart, 2019, p 1259)

The NHS thus has a long and complex history of fundraising and voluntary contributions at the local level. However this chapter focuses on the advent of a new, and explicitly *national* (in this case, UK-wide) mode of fundraising for the NHS during the COVID-19 pandemic.

National NHS fundraising in the COVID-19 pandemic

Charitable funding within the NHS escalated rapidly during the COVID-19 pandemic. The key driver of this shift was NHS Charities Together's Urgent COVID-19 Appeal. NHS Charities Together is an association of around 240 local NHS charities across the UK, which support local NHS organisations with funds to supplement core government-funded services (NHS Charities Together, 2022a). Formerly known as The Association of NHS Charities, the membership organisation gained charitable status in 2008, and rebranded to the current NHS Charities Together in 2019, with a more public-facing strategy (NHS Charities Together, no date). The rebrand included legal changes to the status of the charity:

> I thought well if we're raising the profile and we're trying to raise the profile externally then we need an external way of talking about us. So we gained a brand licence to use that and we renamed ourselves, rebranded in 2019 to NHS Charities Together. We incorporated, because the organisation was unincorporated and therefore to be able to grow and do some of these more external and risky things, we needed to incorporate to be able to mitigate risk to the trustees and to the organisation itself. ... We'd incorporated, so we were now a newly incorporated charity at the beginning of 2020, which we'd done at the end of 2019. We'd got our new brand. (Senior staff member, quoted in Möller and Abnett, under review)

Part of this strategy included a shift towards collective national fundraising appeals, with the advent of a branded fundraising event called the NHS Big Tea, held in 2018, 2019 and 2022 on 5 July, the anniversary of the 'appointed day' when the NHS was created.

At the start of the COVID-19 pandemic, NHSCT launched a dramatically successful fundraising campaign. An online blog by a firm of charity consultants brought in to support the appeal describes a spontaneous 'groundswell of love and support for the NHS' (More Partnership, 2020) in early March 2020, prompting NHSCT to launch an appeal on the day the nationwide lockdown was announced. NHSCT's Chief Executive Ellie Orton is quoted stating 'but we were not a fundraising organisation and we were inundated with 100,000s of enquiries from people wanting to do things for us. ... Our website was overwhelmed' (Brindle, 2020). In a few months, the charity's tiny staff team of four increased to 25, and the appeal eventually raised over £150 million (NHS Charities Together, 2021). While the groundwork for the appeal had been laid in the new strategic direction for the organisation in the years before the pandemic, the shift to a major national appeal was therefore primarily reactive:

> That was a kind of starting point to say there are a group of people out there who will support the NHS as an abstract idea, as a good thing to support. And certainly once we got into the pandemic it became clear that there were lots of organisations and individuals who wanted to support the NHS as a whole rather than a specific hospital because of the challenge they could see that we were facing or that the hospitals were facing. So really things took off in quite an unexpected way, I suppose, certainly in terms of the amount of money that we raised. (Senior staff, quoted in Möller and Abnett, under review)

The contrasting of 'the NHS as an abstract idea' with 'a specific hospital' here is significant. Before 2018, *all* charitable fundraising for the NHS had been led locally by NHS charities, with appeals often focusing on specific hospitals. The first NHS Big Tea fundraiser in 2018 was a major shift away from this approach, which paved the way for the speed of NHSCT's response to the beginning of the COVID19 pandemic. Another interviewee framed the project facing NHS Charities Together in the aftermath of the startling fundraising successes of the pandemic period, as channelling the strength of public feeling for 'the NHS' into something that can be more meaningfully supported:

> The enormous outpouring was for just the NHS as a concept and a loosely understood entity which it's not really. We are an entity, we are a charitable entity and therefore an appropriate source for charitable support, so making the switch in people's mind from a charitable point of view between the NHS and NHS Charities Together is the immediate challenge going forward. (Senior staff, quoted in Möller and Abnett, under review)

Acknowledging that, as argued in Chapter 1, 'the NHS' is far from a coherent organisational entity, this interviewee presents NHS Charities Together as 'an appropriate' organisational vehicle to translate the 'enormous outpouring' for the NHS.

Reconfiguring the NHS as a charitable cause

In the early months of the pandemic, I worked with other researchers to 'capture' fundraising pages for the NHS Charities Together's Urgent Appeal, and then conducted a thematic analysis of the text of 945 fundraising appeals (this analysis is more fully reported in Stewart et al, 2022) created on JustGiving and GoFundMe in the first months of the COVID-19 pandemic, where the recipient was NHS Charities Together's COVID-19 Urgent Appeal. Page captures took place between mid-May and mid-June 2020, during the UK's first national lockdown in response to the COVID-19 pandemic. Accordingly, the data is a snapshot of what we now know to have been the early months of the prolonged COVID-19 pandemic, as people fundraised for NHS Charities Together in response to the new challenge.

Many of the findings of this analysis focus particularly on the COVID-19 pandemic as a moment for British society. In common with other analyses, they tell a story of a moment of profound uncertainty, as national lockdown was declared, schools and workplaces were closed and the government asked us to 'stay home, protect the NHS, save lives'. This was also, for many although not all, a time of boredom, when everything was cancelled and before the digital pivot moved social lives online. These pages demonstrate the experimentation and the improvisation of the exceptional early days of the pandemic, when daily life was suddenly transformed (Erikainen and Stewart, 2020). On the other hand, they are rich with the militaristic metaphors which others have identified as being a significant and problematic feature of the pandemic (Cox, 2020; Olza et al, 2021; Semino, 2021), and which Bivins (2020) has argued has been a feature of discussion of the NHS since its post-war origins. COVID-19, here, is recast as a formidable enemy, and the NHS becomes the army which the population need to back. In this chapter, I mobilise this dataset to specifically explore how members of the public construct *the NHS* as a deserving or worthwhile cause within their fundraising pages.

Fundraising approaches

The pages analysed included a range of sponsored activities and fundraisers, often undertaking a physical challenge. Many of these were 'equivalent' challenges where significant feats, such as climbing Britain's highest mountain Ben Nevis, could be accomplished within contemporary restrictions on being out of the home for 'daily exercise' ('we worked out that if we go up and down our stairs at home 50 times a day (each) for 13 days, we will have climbed the 1345 metres height of Ben Nevis'). One notable subset of pages (around 10 per cent of the total) featured touching stories of children fundraising for NHSCT, often written using children's own (or childlike) words, although all pages had to be created by an adult:

> I'm stuck at home doing home school while a terrible virus out in our world and it's scary. My step dad is recovering from COVID-19 …

I'm raising money in aid of NHS Charities Together/Association of NHS Charities and every donation will help. Once I've hit my target I promise I will shave my hair all off.

More common were runs, bike rides, or 'sit up' challenges, often explicitly referencing that fundraisers had been inspired by Captain Tom Moore's efforts. At least 40 pages explicitly referenced being inspired by Captain Tom Moore: 'If we smash the distance we will not stop – Captain Tom Moore didn't, so neither will we!' The magnitude and persistence of Captain Tom Moore's achievements were often described as a driver of the pages: which accordingly became unusually positive, even perky, by contrast to conventional healthcare fundraising which foregrounds narratives of suffering.

In many of the pages the tales of deservingness which other research has identified as a feature of healthcare crowdfunding (Paulus and Roberts, 2018; Igra et al, 2021; Kenworthy, 2021) were present but inverted.

[Katie] who has Cerebral Palsy and a brain malformation, has been going out on daily walks for her exercise, using her splints and walker. She has gradually managed to increase her distance up to around one mile per walk, which, for her, probably feels like she has run a marathon each day. In these difficult times, following discussion with [Katie], we have decided that it would be a good idea to use her achievements to help others.

In this example, again echoing Captain Tom Moore, the deserving and impressive story is of the fundraiser, whose sacrifice and achievements are foregrounded, rather than the cause. Indeed any detail on the purpose of the fundraising cause somewhat recedes, with only a statement of NHS goodness: 'The NHS is amazing. It is there for us at the most profound moments in our lives, no matter who we are or what we need.'

Indeed, especially among the earliest pages, some bore only a tangential connection to the formal fundraising appeal from NHS Charities Together. These included pages which sought money to make something (face masks, T-shirts with motivational messages, a keepsake like a small sculpture), to be offered to deserving groups (sometimes bereaved families or hospitalised patients, but often healthcare professionals) with any residual funds to be donated to NHSCT. These, we argue, reflect the initially disorganised, somewhat anarchic approach to fundraising (both in terms of a collective understanding of what was needed, and how to meet that need). For example, one page fundraising to give a gift to bereaved families of NHS staff, proposed:

This campaign is asking for your support to make and present [sculptures] to each of their families as a small token of the nations' appreciation. This campaign is entirely not-for-profit, all funds raised will go to the creation of [sculptures] and any surplus will be donated to the NHS Charities Together.

On this page, little focus is placed on any need or desire for the objects, but rather on the virtuousness of the sacrifices made by NHS staff and their families, and the value in repurposing objects 'originally commissioned for a charitable event ... now cancelled'. Pages seeking donations to fund the creation of face masks or even scrubs similarly centred the (COVID-related) untapped skills and capabilities of the fundraiser:

We have the equipment and resources to help the 'volunteer army' manufacture vital PPE for the NHS, fast. As a very small business we will be giving our time, capabilities and people, along with some raw materials – however this is where we will need some help. ... Any money not used for filament and fabric will be donated to NHS Charities Together.

In supporting small businesses or the 'bedroom production' of items, donations were made into something tangible that promised immediate impact at a time of urgent need. Reading them several years later, with better knowledge of technical requirements for COVID-19 Personal Protective Equipment (and indeed scandals about PPE procurement and availability), they seem naïve in the face of the pandemic.

Even as appeals became more standardised over time, most of the pages remained characterised by considerable ambiguity regarding the allocation of funds and their recipients. While the vast majority of pages clearly identified NHSCT as the sole benefactor, some split donations between different charities. Many of the pages did not distinguish between the NHS and the national charity, inaccurately promising that any money would 'be sent directly to the NHS to help in their fight against COVID-19'. Others even implied direct cash transfers – suggesting that the 'fund will go directly to the NHS workers' – when in practice support grants were paid out to local NHS charities with some discretion on how best to meet urgent needs. Some appeals by artists who were financially affected by lockdown restrictions claimed that 50 per cent of the proceeds would go towards the NHS or simply chose a limit, above which all proceeds would be donated. Over time (during the relatively short period of our snapshot), pages became more coherent and purposeful. In this, they were aided by the increasing inclusion of standardised text provided by NHSCT themselves.

The NHS as a cause

As mentioned earlier in the chapter, fundraising pages often positioned NHS staff as soldiers, fighting the virus as an enemy. Reflecting the early days of the UK pandemic, where the population was mostly locked down at home, NHS staff and volunteers are depicted as 'heroes' going *out* to a distant frontline to battle COVID-19:

> Men and women that everyday fight a battle for us and our lives, in and out of hospitals and care homes, while having little in the way of protection for their own health.

> NHS Staff are out there on the frontline fighting it so that we can have our normal lives back.

The location of these perceived battles – at a 'frontline' – is identified as spatially distanced from fundraisers' lives, confined largely to their homes in lockdown. There is a contrast here with UK media narratives of citizen responses identified by Erikainen and Stewart (2020), in which everyone is 'doing their bit' on the home front. Many fundraising pages described the desire to 'do something' in a period where risk was strongly differentiated between NHS staff and other 'keyworkers', and the population at home.

Relatedly, we coded a range of phrases across many of the pages as describing a sense of duty: 'We must all play our part', 'give something back to the NHS', 'they deserve our support' and 'we owe so much'. The frequent use of 'we' and 'our' here mobilised a collective entity. One phrase from the standardised text discussed earlier ('our turn to make sure we look after them, to ensure they can keep doing their vital work') recurred frequently within this code. Within the sense of duty our coding distinguished pages which mobilised a reciprocal sense of duty (in which the desire to fundraise was linked to the level of sacrifice of current NHS staff, and a desire to enable them to keep protecting the population): "Every one of us are relying on the brave people in the NHS and Care sector. Let's put our hands in our pockets and make a difference". In other pages, the duty was more generalised (simply presented as the normatively right thing to do): 'Because not doing something to help would be wrong.' Pages often couched 'doing one's bit' in terms of a baseline of relative helplessness: 'do what I can'.

> To me and you, it may feel like we're not able to do anything, but we can still help from home too.

> Everyone feels pretty helpless at the moment but it doesn't mean we can leave it to others.

Important that we try to help each other out in whatever way we can.

These pages expressed feelings of frustration during periods of self-isolation where symbolic acts, like shaving one's head, were perceived as the only way to help from a distance. Such individual challenges and symbolic acts thus seemed to represent an outlet to challenge intense feelings of anxiety and powerlessness into something creative and productive: "In times like these, where some of us have never felt so distant, it is important to show unity and love. To stand together and support in any way possible, be it humour, creativity, or even just to be a listening ear and a shoulder to cry on." Doing something, here, becomes normatively desirable as a show of 'unity and love' to a 'good cause', but significantly absent a clearly defined goal, or indeed an articulated belief that doing *these* things would significantly aid *that* cause.

In sharp contrast to analyses of conventional healthcare fundraising, in which personal disclosure of suffering, vulnerability and deservingness is the central communicative function of narratives, we encountered relatively few personal experiences of ill-health or loss within these pages. Fewer than 10 per cent of pages were coded as having *any* reference to the fundraiser's personal experience with healthcare, and this included pages where fundraisers described working for the NHS: "I have had the horror of witnessing the strain it has put on all staff first hand whilst myself working as a doctor in intensive care."

Strikingly, most pages which mobilised personal health experiences recounted *past* experiences of (often life-saving and life-changing) healthcare, which were described as demonstrating the importance and deservingness of the NHS:

My personal story is of the NHS saving and rebuilding my life following two catastrophic strokes.

Not many people know this about me but the NHS saved my life. … This is just one example of the amazing work that all doctors and nurses do at the NHS on a daily basis. I'm sure you have your own personal stories of how the NHS has helped you or a family member or friend.

Comparing these narratives to those mobilised within personal fundraisers in existing research demonstrates how measured and positive they are. Fundraisers for the NHS, as well as making less use of their personal experiences, have less need of the 'highly-vulnerable self-disclosures' (Gonzales et al, 2018) which characterise personal fundraising. In effect, NHS fundraisers rely on collective representations to convey the deservingness which individual fundraisers strive to demonstrate individually.

The ontological basis of the NHS as cause – just what is being supported – is an intriguing aspect both of the wider appeal and of the pages which individuals and groups went on to create. Historically, charitable fundraising in the NHS has been highly localised, in that specific organisations (a hospital, for example) have held and fundraised for their own funds. As mentioned earlier, NHS Charities Together's *national* fundraising only began in 2018, and there is thus no real tradition in the UK of donating to 'the NHS' rather than to one's local hospital, or a specific local appeal. Nonetheless, references to 'our wonderful NHS', 'our fantastic NHS' and our 'amazing NHS' were prevalent. Overwhelmingly, fundraisers focused these narratives of gratitude on the NHS workforce, praising their commitment, the risks under which they were working and their sacrifices.

> Imagine having to leave your family to go and work with infected patients, never knowing if you're going to come home with the virus – or in some sad cases, come home at all. It's a huge sacrifice they're making for us and I think we should show all show our appreciation.

Placing potential donors in an imagined position of vulnerability and risk here became a powerful discursive strategy to evoke strong emotional responses, but also feelings of solidarity and moral indebtedness.

Staff were frequently described as heroes, a framing which later in the pandemic would become formalised into a proactive marketing campaign from NHS Charities Together: *Be There for Them* (NHS Charities Together, 2022b). During lockdown, the idealisation of NHS workers as heroes or frontline soldiers can be seen as a way of coping with intense feelings of powerlessness and unequal exposure to risk. Such idealisation of virtue and care typically occurs as a defence mechanism during periods of anxiety, threat or emotional difficulty (Leduc-Cummings et al, 2020). Staff wellbeing is one of the most obvious ways for charitable money to be used in the NHS, given restrictions which exist on charitable money paying for things which should be provided through statutory funding. Many pages drew on the phrase 'above and beyond what the NHS alone can provide' from NHSCT's standardised text, leaving open what constitutes these 'extras'. Unlike findings in both Chapter 5 on campaigning, and Chapter 6 on reviewing service use, relatively few fundraising pages referred explicitly to need generated by *mis*-management or perceived underfunding of the NHS. For example, one recurrent theme was around the provision of Personal Protective Equipment (PPE). A shortfall of quality PPE for health workers, and failings in government procurement of additional stock, became a major political issue as the pandemic unfolded (Oliver, 2021). At this early stage of the pandemic fundraisers more often referred to it neutrally as accentuating the risks staff were taking when they went to work, rather than assigning blame for the lack of PPE available.

As well as a focus on staff wellbeing, fundraising pages also centred a sense of togetherness between NHS and population. This shares some similarities with the function of individual crowdfunders in building social support for people in difficult positions: Gonzales et al note successful individual fundraisers expressing positive benefits from reconnecting with their existing social networks, and building new ones (Gonzales et al, 2018). In the NHS fundraisers, this togetherness suffused many of the pages – with references to 'our' NHS, to 'the community' and even, albeit less frequently, 'the nation'. Sometimes fundraisers involved sponsored, socially-distanced activities to encourage togetherness: for example 'to allow people to come together in song, to feel a part of something bigger in the world and to support one another'. In others, donations are seen as communicating togetherness to NHS staff: 'Let them know the country has got their back', 'we've got this!'. While often fairly generalised, in a handful of pages these pleas for collective togetherness were expressed as a response to the unsettling feeling of one's *usual* societal structures being removed:

> When the corona virus outbreak started, I noticed that a lot of the things we take for granted stopped working. People started dying. I turned to my local authority for info and there was nothing there. … Community is all we truly have and we must support and help each other. … The NHS is amazing. It is there for us at the most profound moments in our lives, no matter who we are or what we need.

The reference to the NHS – a vast, national organisation – here seems almost anachronistic, in a post which refers to intensely localised and non-medical desire for normality.

Conclusion

Beyond the specific practices of fundraising money for the NHS, fundraising money for healthcare is an increasingly prevalent phenomenon. It is facilitated in this by large international crowdfunding platforms, which ease the path of fundraising, while also 'mediating and influencing individual and collective responses to crisis' (Kenworthy et al, 2022). This chapter explores how widespread and familiar modes of appealing for money, and raising it, using digital platforms, were mobilised as an act of love for the NHS in the early months of the COVID-19 pandemic. As it happens, the COVID-19 Urgent Appeal that these fundraising pages supported was exceptionally successful, and seems likely to have formed a critical juncture in the broader landscape of NHS charities (Stewart and Dodworth, 2020; Harris and Mohan, 2021). However this analysis focuses not on the precise sums raised, or their use within cash-strapped NHS organisations, but on how, discursively, fundraisers sought to frame their appeals and render them persuasive.

The uniqueness of the context of this COVID-19 campaign can hardly be overstated. The fear and uncertainty of the early months of the pandemic were pervasive in the UK. I remember anxiously watching a news report from overwhelmed Italian hospitals, and sitting dumbstruck on the sofa as Prime Minister Boris Johnson announced the 'hard' national lockdown, with immediate effect. It is also easy to forget, that in the *first* lockdown, people who were not deemed 'keyworkers' were, to a far greater extent than in subsequent lockdowns, unoccupied: 8.9 million workers were formally furloughed through the Coronavirus Job Retention Scheme on 8 May 2020 (Francis-Devine et al, 2021). It took time for social events and work meetings to 'pivot' online. With the closure of social care, schools and childcare establishments, those with caring responsibilities were far from idle (Özkazanç-Pan and Pullen, 2020). But routines were disrupted, and the success of NHS Charities Together's COVID-19 appeal suggests the opportunity to undertake enjoyable fundraising activities in pursuit of a 'good', if indistinct, cause, was a particularly attractive one during this period of inactivity and existential anxiety.

The peculiarity of this pandemic moment makes the success of NHS Charities Together's COVID fundraising campaign more, and not less, intriguing as a manifestation of public love for the NHS. There were relatively lowered barriers for joining in the fundraising effort (thanks to the formal campaign from NHS Charities Together, and to people having more time at home than usual) as well as the particular psychological benefits (feeling part of something, celebrating togetherness at a time of fear). In the Austrian context, Prainsack (2020, p 128) described 'news media drunk with celebrations of solidarity' as groups went out of their way to support more vulnerable neighbours in the early months of the pandemic. But, she argues, this was an unsustainable phenomenon, based on a protective instinct towards the 'clinically vulnerable' for whom (we had been told) lockdown was necessary to protect, rather than a more enduring recognition of our 'shared vulnerability as humans'. Thus the segmentation of the population whether via differential regulation, or simply within government rhetoric, has deeper sociological consequences (Ganguli-Mitra et al, 2020).

The character of the fundraising pages people created in this exceptional moment is still revealing of *how* Britain loves the NHS. Overwhelmingly, people described their support for the NHS not in the terms of 'patient satisfaction' nor even that of the 'grateful patient' who so dominates US accounts of healthcare fundraising (Collins et al, 2018). The actual 'nuts and bolts' of healthcare were almost entirely absent from the textual and visual content of these pages, beyond the ubiquitous surgical facemasks of stock images of NHS heroes. Rather than the material, embodied everyday work of healthcare, these appeals foregrounded epic, abstract themes around nationhood, heroism, and solidarity. What Dean (2020) describes as 'the good glow' of charitable giving, was coupled with the enduring appeal of 'our' NHS to remarkable effect. This harked back to early political discourse around the NHS in the 1940s, which sought to galvanise a national sense of purpose around the service and positioned it as 'a site for continued patriotic effort and even sacrifice' (Bivins, 2020). 'The NHS' discursively stood in, temporarily at least, for societal commitments, not for a provider of prescriptions, nor operations. The persuasive 'worthy' appeal, such a central and challenging feature of most healthcare crowdfunding pages (Paulus and Roberts, 2018; Kenworthy, 2021), is barely made. Simply put, the cause is 'good'. This speaks, I argue, to the way that the NHS's discursive positioning increasingly unites sub-groups of the population who would often be at odds, if not actively in conflict. The Union Jack branding and the surge in militaristic, World War II narratives (Erikainen and Stewart, 2020) resonates with a centre right and even right-wing segment of the population who would usually deplore 'big state' welfare state commitments (Fitzgerald et al, 2020). And the NHS's vaunted founding principles – universalism, funding through progressive general taxation – continues to engage more left-wing and social democratic constituencies in its defence.

4

Volunteering in the NHS

Volunteering in healthcare is a significant and longstanding public practice in the UK, considerably predating the NHS (Gorsky, 2015). However our knowledge of this diverse and often informal set of practices is, perhaps inevitably given those characteristics, somewhat patchy. A major report in 2013 noted a 'striking lack of information' on the topic (Naylor et al, 2013). This is typical of the wider literature on volunteering in general, with definitional issues alone complicating analysis (Lindsey et al, 2018). The King's Fund used surveys to yield an estimate of around 3 million volunteers in health-related causes in England alone, similar numbers to the whole paid NHS and social care workforces in England at the time (Naylor et al, 2013). Another King's Fund survey, again focused only on England, reported 78,000 volunteers working within acute trusts alone (Galea et al, 2013). A more recent study of community hospitals in England found that these small hospitals had a mean of 24 volunteers each (Davidson et al, 2019; Paine et al, 2019). Data from Healthcare Improvement Scotland reports 2,690 volunteers giving their time across 15 of Scotland's Boards in 2021 alone (Healthcare Improvement Scotland, 2022).

Volunteering in and around healthcare is thus not a singular phenomenon, and the boundary between formal NHS volunteering and third sector volunteering to support health and wellbeing is particularly blurry (Malby et al, 2017). Giving time at the local level, such as in hospitals close to home, has a history before the creation of the NHS and continues on beyond it (Paine et al, 2019; Ramsden and Cresswell, 2019). Sometimes these roles are managed and recruited by a national organisation (such as my own experience volunteering in a hospital café run by the Royal Voluntary Service) and sometimes they are much more informal. In a helpful report, Malby et al (2017) distinguish modes of volunteering: informal and formal; episodic or ongoing; in different types of settings; made up of different activity types. Reported activity types include a remarkably broad range of practices, from helping patients 'navigate' the health system, to participating in research, working in a café or sitting on a committee (Galea et al, 2013). For the purposes of this chapter I set to one side related activities such as timebanking (Glynos and Speed, 2012; Bird and Boyle, 2014;) and peer-led support (South et al, 2012) and focus on roles which can be construed as directly supporting the NHS, rather than a more specific community of interest or identity. This chapter focuses on volunteers' perspectives on NHS volunteering. I begin by reviewing the overlapping and sometimes competing frames through which health-related volunteering is currently valued and promoted in UK policy debates, including in the flurry of NHS branded volunteer schemes which sprang up during COVID. Then, I turn to explore the perspectives of people volunteering in and around the NHS, emphasising the affective and political dimensions of volunteering in healthcare. I draw on a range of data sources: qualitative interviews with people volunteering in the NHS in Scotland, surveys of volunteers commissioned by large organisations (Helpforce and the Royal Voluntary Service), and finally, my own three months spent volunteering weekly in a Royal Voluntary Service café in a Scottish hospital in 2022 (see Chapter 8 for further details).

Valuing volunteering in the NHS: policy frames

Volunteering in the NHS has been promoted both by health policy and by external organisations over the decades. Across this time period, there are varying justificatory frames within this policy area, ranging from 'base imperatives of economic necessity and naïve anti-statism, to loftier impulses, such as the desire to inculcate civic virtues, or to promote individual wellbeing and the formation of social capital' (Lindsey et al, 2018, p 217).

National voluntary organisations have played a key role in coordinating NHS volunteering since its earliest days. The Royal Voluntary Service was created as the Women's Voluntary Services for Air Raid Precautions in 1938 (Mcmurray, 2008). Within a year of its creation, the organisation was working in hospitals with a focus on the war effort, and while it was initially assumed that volunteer numbers would reduce after the Second World War, 'WVS volunteers ... continued to provide their services and expanded on areas such as feeding and fundraising' (Hunt, 2016). Other international organisations also providing volunteers within the NHS include the British Red Cross (Cresswell, 2020) and St John Ambulance. Ramsden and Cresswell argue that, while the Second World War was a high point for volunteering from the Voluntary Aid Societies:

> Just because a new supposed social democratic consensus suggested that the welfare of the individual would now be entrusted to the state, this did not mean that older traditions of voluntaristic self-sacrifice to a greater communal and national good, an instinct and ideology that had recently come to the fore in the war effort, would simply disappear. (Ramsden and Cresswell, 2019, p 529)

Brewis (2013) argues that far from being replaced wholesale by paid professionals, volunteers and voluntary organisations were a central part of the expansion of the welfare state in the 1940s and 1950s.

This co-existence of pre-NHS voluntaristic commitments with state-centric planning continued in the intervening decades. The Ministry of Health issued national guidance for the recruitment and management of volunteers in 1962 (Rochester, 2013). In its 1977 evidence to the Royal Commission on the NHS, the King's Fund stated that the national organisations 'are likely to remain the bulwark of any voluntary activity' (King Edward's Hospital Fund for London, 1977), but also emphasised the need to engage young people and patient groups in volunteering. They called for a greater focus on the organisation of volunteering: 'A decisive lead is called for in this important field and encouragement must be given to the allocation of what must be relatively modest sums when counted against the total budgets of the authorities concerned' (King Edward's Hospital Fund for London, 1977). The report of the Commission itself acknowledged 'the unique and varied contribution made by volunteers to the NHS' (Merrison, 1979) and stated that some training and coordination of volunteers was advisable. Continued financial support of voluntary effort was recommended.

Despite these pleas, the 1980s saw limited policy focus on the potential contribution of volunteering in the NHS. The King's Fund continued to call for investment in volunteer training and support (Pitkeathley, Volunteer Centre, King's Fund Centre and Gay, 1982). The Department of Health scheme Opportunities for Volunteering was created in the 1980s and ran for 30 years, seeking to encourage volunteering of unemployed people through a list of national organisations who acted as National Agents (Department of Health, 2011). The year 2011 saw a new strategic vision for volunteering published by the Department of Health, and the end of the Opportunities for Volunteering scheme (Department of Health, 2011).

In the 2010s, key actors including the King's Fund continued their calls to formalise NHS volunteering in order to maximise the potential benefits to the health system, and a significant new organisation, Helpforce, emerged. In 2013 and then 2018 the King's Fund called for a more strategic approach to volunteering in health and social care (Firth, 2013; Ross et al, 2018), including a call for all Trusts to have a formal volunteering strategy. This followed similar efforts in Scotland, including first the requirement for all Boards to have a Strategic Lead for Volunteering (Feeley, 2008), followed by an additional requirement for an Executive Lead for Volunteering (Leitch, 2019). In promoting more 'strategic' approaches, such moves sought to centre health system demand from a more organic focus on the wishes of those volunteering:

Interviewees described a shift away from supply-led volunteering towards demand-led thinking: 'Not what do volunteers want to do, but where can they make an impact.' Health and care organisations provide a public service, and volunteer co-ordinators are increasingly driven by the question: 'What is the demand?' and 'What is the capacity to support volunteers?' (Malby et al, 2017, p 10)

This quote is from a 2017 report commissioned by the charity Helpforce, which had been created a year earlier by investment banker Sir Thomas Hughes-Hallett with a vision to 'find new ways for individuals and communities to contribute to our healthcare system' (Hanrahan, 2018). Moving beyond calls for NHS organisations to manage volunteering more effectively, this report called for a better approach to volunteering to 'save' the NHS (Malby et al, 2017). It grounded this in an assertion that the NHS had been 'built on voluntary foundations' but that in the decades since it 'developed in a different way, seeking to organise itself by deploying professional knowhow and scientific knowledge alone' (Malby et al, 2017).

Volunteering, in this vision, is a route to (re)humanising healthcare by expanding community roles within the system. Referencing NESTA's People-powered health project (NESTA, 2013), they argue

Actual experience, as described in a series of films which the People-Powered Health team made, is that it can be transformative, changing the power balance between people and professionals. There is also evidence of a huge untapped demand from patients and service users to use their time and human skills to help other people, as long as it is in some way mutual. Nesta calculated that People-Powered Health along these lines would cut NHS costs by at least 7 per cent and maybe up to a fifth. (Malby et al, 2017, p 39)

Thus volunteering is presented as an untapped resource to compensate for deficits in the health system: 'Imagine that health professionals had the time to make everyone feel valued and cared for personally. Imagine there was an infinite resource to provide the kind of informal care that keeps people healthy. Imagine there was enough time' (Bird and Boyle, 2014; see also Ross et al, 2018).

Since the beginning of the pandemic, debates about healthcare volunteering have taken on a more pragmatic, 'emergency response' character. Health-related volunteering flourished following a call for an NHS 'volunteer army' (Tierney and Mahtani, 2020), and a broader range of the population were drawn into 'emergency' volunteering roles (Mak et al, 2021). Across all volunteering areas there is some evidence that these emergency volunteering roles (such as community mutual aid) were a brief flourish, rather than the beginning of a longer-term trend (Acheson et al, 2022). However, in the healthcare context it has added impetus to pre-existing efforts to expand the quantity and effectiveness of NHS volunteering. As I will discuss later in this chapter, this has continued since, with a strong focus on bolstering a healthcare system which many argue is under unprecedented stress, and a series of announcements about an 'auxiliary ambulance service' of volunteers (Taylor, 2022; Warnes, 2022).

In parallel to these developments, there has been a push to promote the benefits of volunteering to volunteers themselves, specifically around transitions to employment, and to make volunteering more inclusive of a broader range of people who might benefit from the opportunity (Kamerāde and Paine, 2014; Stuart et al, 2020; Hogg and Smith, 2021). The association between volunteering and employability is far from straightforward. As Kamerāde and Paine argue: 'Even if volunteering gives people the skills and experience necessary to compete in the labour market, it does not create jobs, solve the childcare problems of unemployed parents or change the prejudices of employers' (Kamerāde and Paine, 2014). Emphasising volunteering as a development opportunity serves several goals for organisations: it might help to recruit more diverse volunteers (shifting away from a stereotype of white, middle class retirees (Matthews and Nazroo, 2021)) with broader benefits for the inclusivity of services; and it might serve to promote volunteering as an employability tool for investment.

Justifying (and ideally quantifying) the value of volunteering in healthcare thus serves multiple political purposes, as well as informing the negotiation of enduring sensitivities with staff and trade unions about job replacement (Handy, Mook and Quarter, 2008; Helpforce and UNISON, 2019). In different ways, each of these visions of volunteering seeks to instrumentalise it for other ends: either to improve (or even 'save') the health system, or to improve the volunteers. This has knock-on effects, encouraging organisations to formalise and document volunteering for the purposes of evaluation (Rochester et al, 2010). It also risks misunderstanding what recruits volunteers. Lindsey et al (2018) distinguish between the sort of instrumental motivations that people might report retrospectively, and the actual routes into volunteering which are more deeply embedded in social context and opportunity. In this chapter I adopt a lens on volunteering as an act of love for the NHS which takes seriously what surveys of volunteers often tell us. That is, people volunteer to do something good, most are essentially altruistically motivated, and pleasure in the social practices of volunteering is key to its appeal for many (Lindsey et al, 2018).

New national schemes for volunteering

Resonating with the upsurge of volunteering around the Second World War, the COVID-19 pandemic, especially in its first year of exceptional public health measures and the country on an emergency footing, has also seen an influx of volunteers both through informal mutual aid and formal organisations. Notably, a series of loosely linked 'NHS branded' schemes have been created in England, including NHS Reservists (NHS England, 2022d), NHS Volunteer Responders (NHS Volunteer Responders, 2020), and NHS Cadets (St John Ambulance, 2021). However it is worth emphasising that schemes emerged out of a pre-pandemic context in which volunteering for 'our NHS' was increasingly promoted. In 2018, the *Daily Mail* launched a Christmas appeal for a 'volunteer army' to give up time for six months to help the NHS. Prime Minister Theresa May stated:

> As a country we are rightly proud of our NHS – it belongs to us all and is there for every one of us in our times of need. It's fantastic that the Daily Mail is encouraging the public to give up their time to help others, be that by visiting patients, picking up their prescriptions or helping the elderly get around hospital. Day in, day out, our doctors, nurses and other healthcare professionals go the extra mile, serving with extraordinary dedication, and making the NHS what it is today. As a Government, we are putting £394m a week extra into the NHS as part of the long-term plan. But we have always been a nation of volunteers. And as this campaign shows, the public can also play a valuable role by offering companionship and support at what can often be a difficult time. (Quoted in Borland, 2018)

Backed by members of the royal family and celebrities such as Joanna Lumley, the campaign reported signing up a remarkable 32,500 volunteers in December 2018 (Pickles, 2019). While the success of the campaign was praised in a 2021 report from the All Party Parliamentary Group on Social Integration (Barrett, 2021), no data has been published on whether everyone who signed up was matched with a volunteering vacancy, nor on the overall value of the campaign in terms of either volunteer or NHS experience.

2020's NHS Volunteers Responders programme was delivered by the Royal Voluntary Service. It included both community support ('Check in and chat', collecting and delivering groceries) and, later in the pandemic, roles such as stewarding at vaccination centres, notably all promoted as 'eas[ing] pressures on NHS staff' (Dolan et al, 2021). The programme worked via a smartphone app (GoodSAM), with the idea that this could allocate one-off, low commitment tasks to a high number of willing volunteers: 'A novel, digital, micro-volunteering programme' (Dolan et al, 2021). One working paper deemed the programme a remarkable success both in scale and in the reported wellbeing of volunteers:

> Three quarters of a million people registered their interest in just four days (NHS, 2020), thus resulting in the largest volunteer mobilisation since World War II. The benefits to vulnerable communities were

considerable: around 165,000 vulnerable people were helped at home during the pandemic from April 2020 to April 2021, with more than 1.8 million volunteering tasks completed. (Dolan et al, 2021, p 3)

However in its early days there was a remarkable mismatch between supply (an upsurge of expression of interest in volunteering) and demand (the NHS's ability to offer tasks). It was reported that in the scheme's first week, it had 750,000 volunteers but a total of 20,000 tasks (Mao et al, 2021).

The NHS Cadets and the NHS Reservists are two other programmes launched since the start of the pandemic. While strongly distinctive programmes, each of these invoke militaristic language in their effort to expand the ways in which members of the public can serve the NHS. Although the rhetoric is redolent of voluntaristic schemes, NHS Reservists are paid and therefore not volunteers. This scheme creates 'a paid, flexible, yet reliable workforce' who are given training and then 'called up' to work for approximately 30 days per year (NHS Careers, 2022). In March 2022, a press release quoted NHS England's Deputy Chief People Officer explicitly emphasised gratitude as a reason to sign up for the scheme and 'stand side by side' with NHS staff:

> The whole country is massively indebted to the hard work of NHS staff over the last two years and there is no better way to show your appreciation than stand side by side with health service colleagues as a reservist. By joining the reservists at this most vital of times, not only will you be stepping up to support your NHS, you will also be joining the most passionate and rewarding teams in the world. (NHS England, 2022d)

NHS Cadets is a youth volunteering programme run by St John Ambulance which launched in 2020 on the 'NHS's birthday' of 5 July (NCVO, 2020). It has a specifically developmental focus compared to the other schemes, including weekly group learning sessions: 'Whilst gaining experience and learning new skills, you'll build your awareness of volunteering in the NHS and benefit your community' (St John Ambulance, 2021).

Propelled by both a sharp increase in societal need, and the requirement to strictly limit physical presence of volunteers in hospitals, the pandemic seems to have stimulated an expansion of these opportunities for people to help in their communities, but specifically in 'NHS branded' schemes with quasi-militaristic rhetoric around service. Notably, in Scotland, Wales and Northern Ireland, while the same flourishing of mutual aid and community efforts was noted (Speed, Crawford and Rutherford, 2022), NHS volunteering post-COVID wasn't 'nationalised' into NHS branded schemes in the same way. NHS volunteering in these parts of the UK remained locally-led by local health boards (NHS Inform, 2022; NHS Wales, 2022), and while national charities who help deliver the English schemes are active in the devolved nations (St John Ambulance, the Royal Voluntary Service, the Red Cross), there is no counterpart to these large national 'branded' schemes above. Speed, Crawford and Rutherford (2022) note that citizen volunteering responses during the pandemic are broadly similar across the four nations. However comparing policy towards across the four nations during the pandemic, they note that the Scottish Government and Welsh Assembly Government's prior focus on collaboration and partnership enabled the more effective mobilisation of volunteers (Speed, Crawford and Rutherford, 2022). In short, the particular NHS branding of calls for volunteering during the COVID-19 pandemic was a distinctively English phenomenon, compared with that in Scotland and Wales.

Exploring volunteer motivation

Disentangling the different elements of volunteer motivation is a complex task (Lindsey et al, 2018), and the expansion of NHS branding and nationalistic 'calls to serve' into what was previously a more fragmented and eclectic landscape of health-related volunteering is an intriguing addition to the mix. As noted, policy interventions have often emphasised the instrumental dimensions of volunteering's 'double benefit' (Hogg and Smith, 2021): how it can serve goals of enhancing volunteers' skillsets and employability, alongside meeting needs within organisations. However, especially during the pandemic context, research which asks volunteers why they give up their time placed much greater focus on affective dimensions, and the power of a 'shared cause':

> Media reports on reasons for volunteering during the COVID-19 pandemic highlights that some people want 'to give back', having received support from the NHS for a previous illness; that it can help individuals feel they are doing something at a time of crisis; or that it enables them to cope with sad accounts they hear every day in the media. These news stories show that people offer to volunteer in anticipation that they might need help in the future, if they get the virus. A sense of solidarity can also be established through joining others in working towards a common purpose. (Tierney and Mahtani, 2020, pp 1–2)

In 2021, RVS commissioned a survey of 1000 adult volunteers from market research organisation PCP. The published report emphasises that 23 per cent of respondents started volunteering to learn new skills and 15 per cent to improve their chances of getting a job (Hogg and Smith, 2021). This supports the report's focus on the 'double benefit' to volunteers as well as to organisations. However the broader results to this question, also stated in the report but much less discussed, show instead a consistent focus on altruism, commitment to a cause and enjoyment as people's reasons for volunteering. Figure 4.1 shows all the possible answers in the survey.

This emphasis on altruistic and social rationales for giving one's time resonates with Lindsey et al's account of the complexities of volunteer motivation (Lindsey et al, 2018). Internationally, it is clear that volunteer motivation depends on context; both the roles available within a healthcare system, and the types of people who volunteer. Portuguese researchers identify learning and development, followed by altruism, as the most pertinent stated motivations for hospital volunteering, especially for young volunteers seeking career recognition (Ferreira et al, 2012). One US study of volunteer Emergency Medical Technicians identified 'desire to help others' and 'learning and development' as the two most commonly cited motivations (Haug and Gaskins, 2012), while an Australian study of hospital volunteers found that 'the primary focus for these contributions is not on narrow self-interest or joint volunteer-organisation interests, but rather on broader interests that transcend the organisation's boundaries' (O'Donohue and Nelson, 2009).

The data presented in Figure 4.1 doesn't allow us to understand the extent to which the NHS acts as a cause that motivates volunteers. Multiple choice surveys don't distinguish volunteering to support the NHS as a cause, from volunteering that happens to take place in the NHS, but for more direct and immediate causes: 'Improving things' by helping a particular patient group, or a local facility such as a community hospital. However, the NHS – with its clinical restrictions on access and reputation for excessive bureaucracy – is in many ways a less obvious candidate for volunteering than, for example, institutions of social care in communities. Davidson et al (2019) identified a perception that community hospitals were 'putting up barriers' to volunteering and under-utilising volunteers as an 'untapped resource'. That, despite this context, there is such a sustained track record of formal healthcare volunteering is intriguing. The rest of this chapter explores contemporary examples of volunteering in and around hospitals to consider how volunteering might both stem from and generate affection for the NHS.

Volunteer perspectives

Local volunteering in NHS services includes activities coordinated by the national organisations and schemes discussed earlier, but also a range of more ad hoc roles. In a study I conducted of hospitals at threat of closure, practices of volunteering ranged from significant, longstanding roles to occasional 'drop in' support at events, and was additionally uneven across the hospitals

Figure 4.1: Reasons for volunteering from survey of 1,000 adults aged 16–65 who are current or recent volunteers

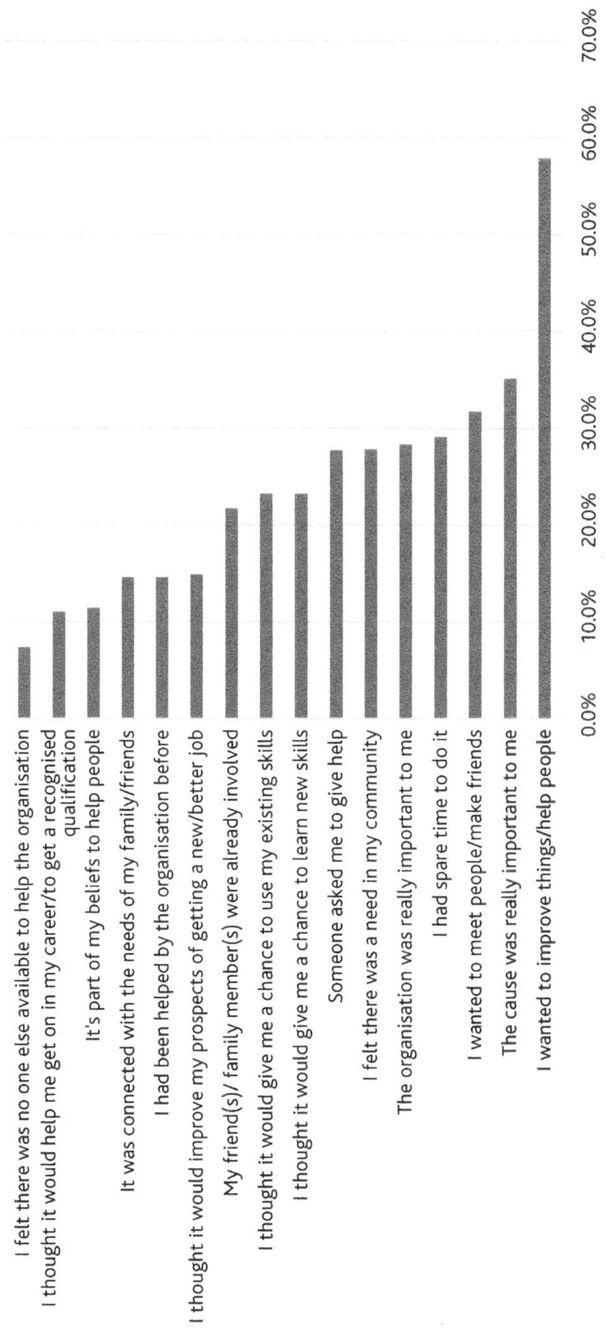

Source: Commissioned by Royal Voluntary Service and summarised in Smith and Hogg (2021)

studied (Stewart, 2019). I spent time researching one community hospital which exemplified the unstrategic, serendipitous nature of much local NHS volunteering, a well-regarded community-run gardening project which had come about when someone with training in therapeutic horticulture moved into the area:

> 'I was doing a talk for somebody else and one of the local councillors approached me and said "do you know about the little patio area up at [hospital 1], it's fallen into disrepair". … So we then set up a steering group, had a couple of interested people, we wrote to the NHS and asked them would it be possible to use the patio area. … We got permission, then we got some funding and raised money to get a summer house … adjacent to where the patio area was, that we could use for indoor work. And then we applied for planning permission to get a ramped area built down to the summer house and we got permission from the hospital to put a disabled toilet inside.' (Catherine, female volunteer, CSO.CS1)

The gardening project, as with similar projects in other hospitals in this study, enhanced the view out of the window for patients in the hospitals. However it also altered the physical grounds in more permanent ways, and integrated into the clinical services provided on site.

> 'Patients from the psycho-geriatric ward, if they were able, would come down and do a one-to-one session with me. Sometimes just the sensory input of being outside and they talked about their previous experiences of having a garden and what they grew in it. Also maybe one or two might come out and watch while the other might do some seed sowing, some transplanting of bud plants etcetera.' (Catherine, female volunteer, CSO.CS1)

Over time, and as patients in the hospital became less physically able to access the garden, some of this work moved inside to the wards:

> 'As a volunteer, [friend's name] and I go in on a Monday morning … and we take garden-related things in, so we do collage work and flower arranging … all related to nature and gardens and get people to talk about what they grow in their garden. … And then after a number of weeks we have a finished product which then the hospital display for us. … The staff are very good at sharing information about the patients with us 'and [we're] certainly good at giving feedback after our sessions if somebody's been very unsettled.' (Anne, female volunteer, CSO.CS1)

Thus a community-led and charitable grant-funded project became integrated as a physical and clinical enhancement to the hospital. Significantly, though, the gardening project had emerged during a period when the hospital's future was up for debate, and continued developing when it was clear that the site would close. The project was designed as far as possible to be portable ('the raised beds can be moved and the summer house can be moved and we can dig out some of the plants and take them elsewhere' [Anne, female volunteer, CSO.CS1]). Thus this emergent enhancement to the hospital, which ticked a number of boxes in terms of community engagement and therapeutic design, was always understood by all concerned as temporary.

Volunteers had devoted time to the gardening project without expectation of a lasting influence, based on their own understanding of local needs. Gardening, and outside spaces, often featured in this study as somewhere where volunteers were given fairly free rein, but also as something that they felt could make a real difference to patient experience. In another community hospital I interviewed a volunteer who had started managing the gardens around the hospital following a loved ones' lengthy stay, and eventual death, in the hospital.

'They leave it entirely up to me which I'm delighted about, and I just treat it as an extension of my other garden. I just go and do what I like, absolutely what I like. A couple of times I've said, any money for a few more plants? And they say certainly – there you are, two hundred pounds, or whatever. So … no, it works; they seem quite happy with it.' (Donna, female volunteer, CSO.CS2)

Hospital outdoor spaces thus offered somewhere volunteers could shape and have ownership of, at one remove from the tighter clinical management of indoor spaces.

Other kinds of NHS volunteering that seemed to have potential for similar levels of autonomy were the 'committee work' that I researched in Scotland (Stewart, 2016). In that book I recounted observing a meeting of a 'Public Partnership Forum' in Scotland in 2010, where a member of NHS staff came along to one meeting to talk about the Board's Investing in Volunteers award. This is an example of the efforts I mentioned earlier to formalise and document NHS volunteering in order to 'improve' it. The member of staff began her presentation with: 'You probably don't see yourself as volunteers, but the public involvement you are doing is volunteering.' In our subsequent interview, one very vocal member of the Forum disputed this: 'We're not volunteers. … All volunteers with the NHS have sort of managers, and people who organise them and what-not. Nobody organises me. Nobody tells me what to do, where to go, when to be there for. We're totally different' (Thomas, PPF member, quoted in Stewart, 2016, p 49). This member distinguished himself from 'the volunteers' on the basis of his specific knowledge and expertise, his role within an external group, and his autonomy and independence, and the fairly ill-defined role of the Forum enabled that for him. His priority was using his expertise on disability to advocate for improvements within the Board. Most members of the Forum, though, had a much more traditional volunteering outlook: 'It's going back to the original idea of joining the NHS as a volunteer ... I thought ... I'd like to do something to sort of show that I'm not completely just sitting back and just getting benefits' (James, PPF member, quoted in Stewart, 2016, p 47). Opportunities to help with public-facing health information and promotional activities, such as hand hygiene stalls in hospital entrances, were welcome for most of the Forum members, who were glad to be helpful. However they sat uncomfortably with more activist members' desire to make change in the NHS organisation, rather than in the broader population.

Increasingly formalised and strategic approaches to volunteering, in well-intentioned pursuit of the 'double benefit' (Hogg and Smith, 2021) and in a context where safeguarding is an appropriate priority, do have tradeoffs in terms of the appropriate level of autonomy for volunteers. This will suit some volunteers more than others. In one hospital case study, a very longstanding volunteer reflected on how her role had fluctuated over the years as different management came in, some with more rigid views on appropriate volunteer contributions:

'We did get quite restricted, we used to be far more involved hands on in the hospital than we are now, because it depends who's in charge whether they want that, do they want volunteers, d'you want just people dropping in. When there used to be daycare there I would've been in the hospital, the day room at least once a week if not twice a week just, you know, I knew all the people and then you would've been bringing things in, you would've been bringing things in for the fly cup[1], you'd of been doing the shopping for the bits and pieces. And then when the daycare finished that was a big change for us, so we didn't feel so involved maybe after that.' (Linda, female volunteer, CSO.CS2)

In this community hospital, an innovative community-led daycare service (see Stewart, 2021) had closed when NHS management decided it constituted social and not medical care. The volunteers had shifted their energies towards supporting wellbeing in the broader community and fundraising for the hospital from the outside.

---

[1] 'Fly cup' is a Doric term for a cup of tea, often along with a sweet treat such as a biscuit, commonly used in the North-East of Scotland.

The argument put forward in Malby, Boyle and Crilly (2017) that volunteers can 'humanise' healthcare, by providing a caring touch, has been evident across my research on community action in the NHS. In the RVS café, I had originally assumed the primary contribution was commercial: I would volunteer in the café, which would increase its profits through not paying staff, and the money would help the cause. The café was emblazoned with large signs in the RVS brand colours: 'Buy here, give back' and 'everything you buy here will support your NHS and local communities'. This is indeed part of the model, and when unhappy customers complained about the price of items in the café we would reply, breezily, 'it's all for charity!' When the complaint came from NHS staff using the café, volunteers might mutter 'it all goes back to them, anyway'. Awkwardness around pricing wasn't uncommon in my experience volunteering in the café. While the café wasn't making profits for a distant company, like the Costa franchise in another local hospital, the nearest shop where inpatients could go to buy something to eat or drink at supermarket prices was some distance away. Daily spending in the café would add up for regular visitors, and alongside snacks and light meals, we sold large bottles of juice and packets of biscuits clearly intended to be brought to the bedside. As a new volunteer, I found the moments when someone couldn't afford what they had intended to buy awkward and difficult to navigate. The mission of 'supporting the NHS and local communities' felt, in these moments, peculiarly detached from the patients and staff standing at the till.

What became clear over time was that the financial rationale for the café, and for the unpaid labour of volunteers within it, was only one of the contributions we made to the hospital. The café, and therefore volunteering within it, served a broader range of 'goods' for the NHS. Perhaps most notably, it was a space of warmth and community where patients, carers and staff received cheer along with their scone or coffee. In some cases this was jovial, with long-running jokes, or compliments between café volunteers and customers. On a sideboard there were always thankyou cards displayed, dropped in by patients or carers as they were leaving after discharge, and often mentioning the 'friendly smiles' of volunteers. Volunteers often stood and chatted with people as they waited for their patient transfer pickup by the door. These moments of kindness and sociability resonated with the accounts of volunteering I heard in community hospitals: "we just do welcome packs, we do the trolley that sort of thing, and a bit of entertainment, and involve people where we can" (Helen, female volunteer, CSO.CS2).

Catering activities here serve broader purposes of connection which go well beyond the sustenance of what the café or trolley sells. The hospital I volunteered in employed paid staff at the entrance, whose role included welcoming people, handing out facemasks and offering directions. This had been a COVID-19-era innovation, and there were rumours in the hospital that if the role was to be retained as the pandemic eased, that the paid jobs would be replaced by volunteers. Such ostensibly low skilled posts are obvious candidates for volunteering (Handy, Mook and Quarter, 2008), but can be a significant intervention in a patient's experience of the hospital.

While not under-estimating the cumulative value of occupying quasi-clinical spaces with humanity and humour, the café also served this purpose during more difficult moments. Sometimes, breaking the daily routine of joviality, it was a space for people to regroup amidst tragedy. One day I got chatting to a customer as I delivered her coffee to her table. She looked tired and, out of the blue, explained she was waiting for a family member, in the aftermath of a traumatic and sudden bereavement. I experienced it as a startling jolt among the mundane, comfortable business of preparing the café for closing, and it occupied much of my fieldnotes for that shift: 'It was so shocking. Every now and again you remember how much sadness is happening in the building.' We gave the customer a free Danish pastry with her drink, since we were closing shortly and they couldn't be sold the next day. It felt utterly futile, of course, and it surely won't have dented the horror of her day. But the particular potential of volunteers to offer moments of human connection can make a difference when we find ourselves in the machine of a modern hospital. As noted in one report: 'Frontline staff clearly appreciate that volunteers can bring additional human kindness into busy hospital life – often by carrying out the smaller, non-clinical actions, such as providing personal and emotional support that staff do not always have time for, which in turn provides staff with more time for clinical care' (Ross et al, 2018). It is important to note the normalisation of a healthcare system being too under-resourced for staff to provide 'personal and emotional support'. Offering personal and emotional support are core to patient experience, but also have a role in staff fulfilment and wellbeing. Nonetheless, research clearly suggests that healthcare volunteers can play a significant and potentially transformative role by offering their time to listen to and support patients.

Volunteering is also a space for, for want of a more intellectual sounding term, fun, for volunteers themselves. Rochester (2013) terms this 'conviviality', and argues it has been neglected from discussions of volunteering. Lindsey et al (2018) describe this as relating to 'triggers' for volunteering, rather than straightforwardly a feature of individual motivation with which people self-identify, but the RVS survey in Figure 4.1 does list 'meeting people or making friends' fairly high. A notable finding of hospital case studies was the virtuous circle of having a committed group of volunteers, who others wanted to join.

'I guess it stems back from … I mean, I guess they're a nice bunch of people, and there's a social aspect to it as well. And I guess, people, you get a sense of satisfaction from knowing that you're doing a good job, and trying to benefit the community. And also, team work, I mean, everybody, whenever they have an event, so many people, whether they're actually on the committee, or whether they're just volunteers who say, yeah I'm gonna come along and help you out at this event.' (Ryan, male volunteer, CSO.CS2)

When volunteering had wound down, committed volunteers described the loss of social connection with sadness.

The enjoyable social element of volunteering took me by surprise during my time at the RVS café. I began quite quickly to genuinely look forward to chatting with the other volunteers and the regular customers, and the silly running jokes that spring up among a team.

> Another week of being really happy to go. I don't know if I look forward to it, but it's such a pleasant change from the usual stresses of work (and stress levels have been quite high about work, all in all). Immediate, easy, pleasant. Already feeling a bit sad about giving it up. (Fieldnotes from volunteering, 2022)

In stressful parts of the academic term, the contrast between my isolated and pressured work alone in my home office, and the sociable ease of the café, with immediate task accomplishment, was stark: 'Last shift! Had a horrible teary morning at work and was in a rush for shift. Such a relief to get into the calm routine of it. And glad to see the other volunteers for a gossip' (fieldnotes from volunteering, 2022). The contrast here was surely increased by what academic work has become during the pandemic: in times gone by my colleagues would have provided at least some gossip and interaction in the coffee room or by the printer. Nonetheless the sheer enjoyment of the 'weak ties' (Lindsey et al, 2018) created by regularly working alongside people I would not usually get to know was a central plank of my volunteering experience, and is rarely mentioned in policy discussion of volunteering in the NHS.

Ironically, another facet of why people volunteer which is relatively neglected in literature seeking to instrumentalise volunteering, is related to 'duty'. This is a somewhat mercurial motivation, in that as well as being unpaid, the 'non-binding' nature of volunteering is key to what differentiates it from work. And yet in case studies I have repeatedly encountered people who volunteer in hospitals due to a sense of duty. Sometimes this related to a pragmatic sense of putting into a local institution to get back, as one interview joked about a closing hospital: "My parents and my brother live down that way so they used to volunteer at the hospital, and I think they used to do that in advance of essentially using it and now they're not going to get the quid pro quo!" (Caroline, female resident, CSO.CS1). Relating to broader discussions of 'being asked' to volunteer (Lindsey et al, 2018), some volunteers describe the invitation as demonstrating the necessity of the activities, and therefore of a duty to step up:

> Enjoying it is not the word. It's something that people need to do. That's how I see it. They wouldn't come in and send me the letters to come and interview me, to put me on the committee, if there wasn't somewhere along the line I was going to be able to, thought I maybe could give something. (Mary, PPF member, quoted in Stewart, 2016, p 47)

Commitment to and gratitude for the NHS often featured highly in these accounts: 'A desire to try and put something back in, you know, to the service I'd had so much from' (James, male PPF member, quoted in Stewart, 2016, p 40).

Conclusion

Volunteering in healthcare is far from a uniquely British phenomenon, but its recent history within the NHS has some intriguing dimensions which justify its inclusion as a practice of care and contestation. Internationally, the availability, nature and formality of available volunteer roles varies by health system context, and comparisons are rendered problematic by the difficulties of robust data on what is an ephemeral phenomenon taking place in highly distinctive health systems (Lindsey et al, 2018; International Labour Organization, 2021). However, research from other countries suggests a series of consistencies and differences between volunteering in different health system context. In the US, volunteers in hospitals are considered 'ubiquitous' (Pickell, Gu and Williams, 2020). Canadian research argues that healthcare volunteering has bucked the trend of an overall reduction in volunteer hours since 2000, and attempts to produce a cost-benefit analysis of volunteering in Toronto area hospitals; claiming 'a return on investment of 684%' (Handy and Srinivasan, 2004). A series of Portuguese studies argues more modestly that there is good evidence that volunteers can improve patient experience of hospitals (Tavares, Proença and Ferreira, 2022).

In the examples of healthcare volunteering discussed in this chapter, the affective and the political dimensions loom large. This supports Rochester's (2013) contention that policy and scholarly discussions of volunteering neglect what he terms expressive behaviours, rather than instrumental goals. Volunteering in the NHS is rooted in the cultural and political status of the healthcare system. With the possible exception of volunteering for current or prospective NHS staff (see for example Mak et al, 2021), volunteering within the NHS is as often concerned with a belief that healthcare in the UK is a cause to support, than with the individual benefits that might stem from it.

That has a number of implications. It asserts that healthcare is a societal good, and not a service to be requested and received from remote professionals. It emphasises the low technology, 'human' aspects of healthcare and their importance in how people engage with and experience health services. And it requires attention to aspects of volunteer matching and management (Malby, Boyle and Crilly, 2017; Hogg, quoted in Miller, 2020) that can be underplayed by quasi-militaristic mass campaigns to recruit NHS volunteers.

In a sense the pandemic became a moment of significant opportunity for the promotion of volunteering in the NHS, including by organisations whose charitable aims are served by tapping into Britain's love for the NHS. As shown earlier, the momentum for volunteering as a solution to a cash-strapped NHS, especially in providing human connection for patients, had been growing well before the pandemic (NESTA, 2013; Malby, Boyle and Crilly, 2017). The *Daily Mail*'s remarkable mobilisation of tens of thousands of volunteers in 2018 suggests that public appetite for time-limited volunteer roles in the NHS is significant, but also that the NHS might struggle to make use of it. The increasing national branding of campaigns for volunteers in England is an intriguing development. The pandemic brought physical restrictions on presence in hospitals and for some, an intense desire for social connection. However the continuation and adaptation of these schemes, and indeed their prominent placement on organisational webpages, suggest that they have ambitions to continue their expansion of a particular vision of volunteering in the NHS. Here, they join the realms of other innovations in which the NHS brand is expanded beyond a narrow definition of healthcare delivery: notably social prescribing and the rollout of 'link workers' in General Practice (Tierney et al, 2020). Such activities do indeed, as Malby Boyle and Crilly (2017) celebrate, dissolve the artificial boundaries between formal and informal care, and between health and social care, in generative ways. But they also superimpose processes onto what might previously have been more serendipitous and flexible engagements and expand a particular formulation of the NHS brand into social and community domains in new ways.

5

Campaigning for the NHS

This chapter explores public campaigns which are oriented around 'the NHS', focusing on them as practices of care and contestation for the healthcare system. This framing of public campaigning departs significantly from a well-established mainstream within contemporary UK health services research (Jones, Fraser and Stewart, 2019), in which public mobilisations around health systems are frequently understood as irrational, and essentially unhelpful obstacles to the 'modernisation' of the NHS. Campaigns to save the NHS, whether through actual demands or more recent 'shows of support', are now common features of public life in Britain. This was not always the case: in important work, historian Jenny Crane (2019) has traced the transformation of public campaigning in and around the NHS, arguing that from the 1960s campaigns were overwhelmingly local and oriented to 'saving' local hospitals earmarked for closure following the 1962 Hospital Plan (see also Jones, 2015), before the emergence of national campaigning in the 'new welfare politics' of the 1980s. This included London Health Emergency's 'Hands off our NHS' campaign, in response to the 1989 White Paper 'Working for Patients'. Crane argues that from the 1980s onwards, response to Thatcherite reforms to the NHS included new tactics of providing and analysing information about healthcare, and new organisational actors in civil society. As well as this broader historical context, NHS-related activism takes place in, and intersects with, the growth of condition-focused patient activism in contemporary health systems (Brown and Zavestoski, 2004; Rabeharisoa, Moreira and Akrich, 2014; Epstein, 2016). We know that social identities shape and are, in turn, shaped by this patient activism, as well as understanding how patient organisations work within and through biomedical research to deliver 'evidence-based activism' (Rabeharisoa, Moreira and Akrich, 2014). In this chapter, I explore the distinctiveness of NHS campaigning at local and national level, reflecting on both the uneasy evocations of 'the NHS' as singular and special, but also on the unusually preservationist (rather than reformist) goals of these campaigns.

This chapter explores two interlinked contemporary forms of activism in the UK context, oriented specifically to 'saving' the NHS. In these, patient identities are present and often mobilised, alongside distinctively public identities to save 'our' NHS as a core part of the British welfare state. I begin by analysing web materials produced by two current campaigns: the 'Keep our NHS Public' campaign, a non-party political campaigning organisation launched in 2015; and 'Your NHS Needs You', a campaign against the 2021 Health and Care Bill. I analyse web materials – including petitions, 'explainer' text and celebrity endorsement videos – to assess how the NHS is constituted as a vulnerable, beloved object in these campaigns. Then, drawing on extensive qualitative data from studies of campaigns to 'save' local hospitals in the 2010s, I explore the activist practices through which members of the public seek to influence local configurations of the NHS. In this, I investigate how 'the NHS' functions as a signifier and object of contention within debates about local hospitals. That is, campaigners must navigate a landscape in which 'the NHS' is both the (local or regional) managers proposing the reconfiguration of a hospital and the hospital itself (Carter and Martin, 2018). Meanwhile, for change-oriented managers, local facilities become a threat to the sustainability of 'the NHS', and hospital closures are seen as necessary in order to protect 'the NHS'. While notionally distinct, and targeting different decision-making authorities, it should be noted that national and local campaigns often intersect. Indeed, Keep our NHS Public is a membership organisation made up of 70+ local campaigns, mostly oriented to saving hospitals. Thus, while different in modality, goal and target, this chapter argues that these campaigns share significant precepts: in the context of the book, caring for the NHS *through* contestation.

Introducing the national campaigns

Your NHS Needs You, a campaign against the 2021 Health and Care Bill (now the Health and Care Act 2022), describes itself as 'a group of doctors, nurses, campaigners, researchers, academics and entertainers working together with DiEM25 to defend the NHS'. At the bottom of the campaign webpage they display logos of 13 organisations, with Diem25 and Unite the Union as the leaders of the campaign. Diem 25 describes itself as a pan-European progressive movement seeking to democratise the EU (for more on Diem25 specifically, see De Cleen et al, 2020). Other organisations include a social enterprise providing counselling and psychotherapy (The Farringdon Practice); We Own It, a campaign to protect public services; The People's Assembly, a national campaign against austerity; Disabled People Against Cuts; the Peace & Justice Project, founded by former Labour Party leader Jeremy Corbyn; the Public and Commercial Services Union; and Every Doctor (a doctor-led campaign for a 'better' NHS).

Keep our NHS Public has existed since 2015, campaigning to 'reverse the privatisation and commercialisation of social care and to call for health and social care services to be publicly funded, publicly provided and accountable provision'. The key focus of the Keep Our NHS Public website was opposition to the Health and Care Bill (now Health and Care Act 2022). The campaign website includes a page of analysis from academics and less-precisely-defined experts, a page of 46 celebrity videos of actors, comedians and entertainers describing their support for the campaign, and details of the parliamentary petition, which (while not preventing the confirmation of the Bill into law) gained 137,713 signatures in the six months it was open. While there is a left-wing emphasis to much of the content and especially the people listed as endorsing the campaign, Keep our NHS Public declares itself a non-party political membership organisation. Members represent over 70 local health campaign groups. Its website lists both national and local 'affiliate' organisations, which include campaign groups (Health Emergency, Doctors in Unite, Doctors for the NHS), journalists (Open Democracy) and other campaigning membership organisations (the Socialist Health Association). The Keep Our NHS Public website includes multiple petitions to Parliament: one, on COVID mitigations and access to testing, signed by over 425,000 people, and another, calling for the Health Secretary to Rebuild the NHS (#endthecrisis), signed by 22,836.

Both Keep our NHS Public and Your NHS Needs You are non-partisan but nonetheless visibly aligned to left-wing party politics. Former Labour Party leader Jeremy Corbyn is listed as a Patron of Keep our NHS Public as 'a committed supporter of a publicly owned and run NHS', as is Green Party MP and former party leader Caroline Lucas. Both of these politicians, along with a number of other left-of-centre Labour Party politicians, also provide celebrity videos for Our NHS Needs You. Both campaigns are focused on the NHS in England only, given their focus on specific reforms to the structure and organisation of care in that country. An additional aspect of note is the extent to which these campaigns present themselves as coalitions of health professionals, patients and members of the public. Compared to earlier campaigns Crane has researched in the NHS, this is a distinctive feature of this political activism in the 2010s, presumably linked to a UK Government which is widely perceived as being unsupportive of the NHS in general.

In both cases I analysed key pages from the campaign website which included discussion of what is valuable about the NHS, and what threatens the NHS. In the case of Your NHS Needs You, I also analysed transcripts of the 'celebrity videos' featured on the page, and widely shared across social media. These videos are short (less than two minutes each), straight-to-camera discussions of what the NHS means to the individual, some discussion of the threats it currently faces and a call to action, starting with a request to viewers to visit the campaign website. These don't appear to be scripted or professionally-produced videos: several of the celebrities joke about how unprofessional their camera work is or background noise from their families. Occasionally repeated turns of phrase, for example private organisations being 'embedded' in the NHS, suggest that celebrities have engaged with the wording of the campaign materials, but the videos are overwhelmingly personal, and characteristic of the speaker's idiosyncrasies. The 46 celebrities include actors, comedians, writers, campaigners and politicians (a full list of these is in Chapter 8). All the elected politicians would be considered left-wing (for example Jeremy Corbyn, Bell Ribeiro-Addy, Caroline Lucas, Yanis Varoufakis), and while the range of celebrities is perhaps less obviously aligned to *party* politics, it is fair to say that the list remains overwhelmingly composed of people who would be considered left-wing in contemporary Britain. It includes a number of people who in Britain are also referred to as 'national treasures' (an epithet also accorded to the NHS on occasion) including Stephen Fry, Michael Rosen and Jo Brand. It is also noticeable that the list is gender balanced, and, by UK media standards, fairly diverse. Two of the videos feature celebrities with disabilities. Six of the 46 videos are from visibly Black and minority ethnic celebrities at a point when around 85 per cent of the UK population are White (Coates, 2021). From the outside, it is difficult to assess the extent to which this diversity is a result of deliberate strategy on the part of the campaign or is happenstance.

In selecting these two national campaigns, I'm mindful of the risks of selection bias. Appeals to welfare nationalism – claiming aspects of the welfare state are specifically *national* achievements, linked to national identity (Béland and Lecours, 2005) – are often embedded within left-wing health politics around the NHS (Fitzgerald et al, 2020; Cowan, 2021). Campaigns of mass mobilisation related to the NHS as a whole are less common in right-wing politics. A key exception is within the various feuding branches of the Brexit 'Vote Leave' campaign, when claims about putative financial savings from leaving the EU being used for the NHS were famously painted onto a campaign bus (for a broader analysis of the NHS's role within that campaign, see Fitzgerald et al, 2020; Stanley, 2022). Even here, though, 'the NHS' operated more as a symbol of where such savings could be reallocated. The campaign materials contained no substantive defence of, let alone proposal for the health system. The only leaflet on the archived Vote Leave website which focuses on the NHS simply states: 'Every week politicians send £350 million of our money to the EU. That's enough to build a new hospital every week. It's almost 60 times more than the amount we spend on our NHS Cancer Drugs Fund' (Vote Leave, 2016). The header of the leaflet features a 'Save our NHS' logo on the header of the leaflet, but no further suggestions for saving it are elucidated. A more detailed briefing produced by the Vote Leave Take Control campaign contains more content, but is still overwhelmingly focused on the putative harms of the EU, such as the European Working Time Directive, and the risks of European trade deals infringing on the NHS: 'If we remain in the EU it will become ever harder to keep the NHS in public hands' (Vote Leave, 2015). In broader public discourse during the Brexit campaign period, the NHS was often linked with racist and imperialist themes. However, reflecting the 'dog whistle politics' of the time (Madden and Speed, 2017), this is less evident from those 'official' campaign materials which remain public. In these, the NHS functions as an empty signifier for British exceptionalism, and campaign materials fail to populate it with an account of the NHS's value. Accordingly, this chapter focuses on more substantial campaigns, which have the added advantage of offering a post-pandemic view of threats to the NHS.

Constructing the NHS in national campaigns

The campaigning webpages articulate a sense of the threats facing the NHS, both in terms of what is to come (why the Health and Care Bill 2021 needs to be opposed) and what has already been diminished. The threat of American corporations is presented as both already embedded in the NHS, and at risk of being further escalated by new proposals. The US health system is presented as the inspiration for reforms that the government is proposing: 'Ushers in American-style Integrated Care Systems (ICSs) ... independent regional bodies initially named Accountable Care Organisations (ACOs) like their American counterparts'. Indeed the Health and Care Bill 2021 is presented as actually handing control of the NHS to these US companies: 'Private corporations and American health insurers will control NHS budgets and receive financial incentives to cut and deny care for profit'. Campaign pages demonstrate a deep appreciation for the ways in which the NHS has *already* been depleted, both by underfunding, but also by substantive changes. Specifically, Keep our NHS Public are forthright on the introduction of additional migrant charges and the increased policing of charging for people deemed overseas patients: 'These charges are an attack on our communities and the basic principles of the NHS.'

On the whole, the video contributions from celebrities focus more on the value of the NHS than specific threats to it. The criticism of policy or calls for reform that Crane (2022) has identified as prevalent in 1980s NHS activism, are notably absent. There are multiple references to the self-evidence of the lovability of the NHS as shared knowledge among an imagined community of listeners: 'I know that you all love the NHS as much as I do' (Kiri Pritchard-Maclean), and 'Our wonderful, beautiful, much-celebrated NHS. You know what it is' (Ben Bailey-Smith).

The campaign webpages echo the sentiment, as though the goal is not to convince readers, but rather to articulate or emphasise something that readers will already, in their bones, know: 'We know how important the NHS is for all of us.' Likewise, petitions recursively refer to surveys of public attitudes to the NHS, arguing that the NHS must be defended because it is valued: 'Surveys of public opinion show the vast majority are in favour of a publicly funded and provided service, paid for through general taxation, free at the point of use and providing comprehensive services.'

One video, from outspoken Scottish comedian Frankie Boyle, flags the elephant in the room among all these common-sense statements of the healthcare system's merits. 'Of course I support the NHS. Everybody supports the NHS, or says they do. And everyone went out and clapped on a Thursday during lockdown' (Frankie Boyle).

Boyle here gestures to the ease with which people can declare their support for the NHS, and hints at a potential gap between statement and sentiment. The functions of these statements about how *everyone* loves the NHS, and their relative lack of substance, can be seen as not merely making a claim about the NHS as a good thing, but going further to suggest that some undefined 'we' *all* agree that the NHS is a good thing. The lack of detail offered in these extracts, the lack of connection to a reason why the NHS is beloved, only reinforces the fact not just that the imagined viewer knows, but that they *should* know. A counter view would require not only disagreement from the reader or viewer, but would be a self-exclusion from the easy, reassuring 'we'; from the 'vast majority' of Britain (Cowan, 2020).

Beyond the NHS as 'a good thing', multiple references go as far as personifying 'the NHS'. Referring to 'the appointed day' on which the NHS came into being (Sheard, 2011), Joe Lycett remarks wryly: 'I share a birthday with it so I feel like we're kindred spirits'. This reflects a shift in which recent 'NHS birthdays' have become increasingly *public* affairs. NHS Charities Together have promoted the 'Big Tea' fundraiser since the 70th birthday in 2018 (NHS England, 2022a), and in 2021, the British Medical Journal reported a 'service of commemoration and thanksgiving' was held to celebrate the Service's 73rd birthday at St Paul's Cathedral in London (Gerada, 2021). Setting aside for one moment the significance of the confluence of church, state and cultural tropes ('a nice cup of tea') that the NHS's birthday has come to represent, the transformation of an albeit significant day of legislative change into a 'birthday' celebration also suggests an ontological shift in understanding of what the NHS is towards something singular and foundational. This resonates with the rise of 'RIP NHS' placards on protest marches from the 1980s onwards (Crane, 2019). Campaign materials reflect this: 'The NHS is the beating heart of this country" (Vicky McClure); 'it's our national treasure' (Shami Chakrabarti). The NHS is cast as a dependable and persistent force for good that 'saved the people I love most in the world' (Kiri Pritchard-McLean). Describing her father ('a walking case study of things that can go wrong with a human'), Pritchard-McLean continues: 'Even when his nearest and dearest give up on him the NHS keeps fighting for him.' The process by which a healthcare system, a vast and complex set of organisations, people and material objects, can 'fight' for a patient, requires it to be condensed into a knowable, and loveable, entity.

Beyond these declarative actions to simplify the scale of the NHS and appeal to everyone's shared love for it, the substantive content of the videos and campaign webpages analysed articulates three distinct, interlinked strands of the NHS's value: gratitude for care received; recognition of the health benefits across society; and finally, the NHS as a source of pride in British identity. To turn first to the expressions of gratitude for care received, these are the overwhelming majority of the transcripts from the celebrity videos. Each person relates one, or a number of examples of care they or their loved ones have received in the NHS. Often, these are life-saving or life-altering tales of medical heroism: 'The doctors came running in and saved her and the baby' (Saffron Burrows). This sort of story explains what one video refers to as a 'visceral connection to the NHS' (Russell Brand), to which several of the videos refer. Stories of personal experience sometimes emphasise the clinical sophistication of the NHS, as when Romesh Ranganathan states he had confidence his family received 'the best care possible'. But more often, stories centre non-clinical aspects of care: that is, the 'devotion' (Barry Gardiner), 'kindness' (Brian Eno) and patience shown by staff. Lemn Sissay's tale is perhaps the best example of how tales of experience locate vital care in the NHS, without a focus on the medical aspects of that care:

'From the ages of 12 to 18 I was in children's homes in the local government and I was never hugged I was never held. It occurs to me that the only time that I was touched with care and with attention was once every six months at my NHS clinic.' (Lemn Sisay)

This poignant example illustrates the way in which NHS continuity functions in these narratives of value. Given that emergency care is not specific to the NHS – that is, other approaches to financing and organising healthcare in high income countries would *also* involve doctors rushing in to save a life in an emergency situation – the characteristic of care most distinctively attributed to the NHS in these campaigns is its reliability as a safety net for society.

Other stories shared are overtly funny, especially where children are concerned:

'It was the uh institution that rehydrated me when I was two years old and had gastroenteritis (I really did eat some weird soil when it was a child) ... and also when I was shocked by a toad and fell over and then bumped my chin on a piece of wood, a sandpit which also cut open my chin.' (Robin Ince)

But, as Ince continues, even these light-hearted anecdotes segue seamlessly into more startling ones: 'And it's the institution that when my mother was in a catastrophic car accident that they cared for her while she was in a coma' (Robin Ince). This range of care experiences – from everyday bumps to traumatic events – across the scope of the health system is explicitly flagged by some of the videos. Emma Kennedy emphasises the 'mundane' role of the NHS in daily life:

> 'So a lot of people are probably going to be telling you stories about how the NHS saved their lives and the NHS do save lives they save lives on a daily basis but I love the NHS for all the more mundane things that they do for us. that they are the the the comfort blanket for when you've got a sore throat or a chesty cough … they're also there for, for the sprained wrists the sprained ankles and all those times that you need an embarrassing cream.' (Emma Kennedy)

Several of this list of minor complaints are, ironically, the subject of public information campaigns encouraging people *not* to seek medical attention for them, but here they are presented as part of the country's 'comfort blanket'. Relatedly, Shappi Khorsandi invokes the shared human experience of embodiment: "Here's why I love the NHS. It's a very simple reason. I am made of flesh and blood. I get ill, my loved ones get ill and they need health care" (Shappi Khorsandi).

A second theme is the recognition of the NHS as a means of meeting not just one's personal healthcare needs but those more broadly distributed across society: as one campaign webpage puts it 'we all need health and social care at some time in our lives, but the unlucky ones need more'. Evoking Bevan's (2010) *In Place of Fear*, Jonathan Ross describes the NHS as giving 'a great sense of reassurance and happiness to me'. This recognises both that one can feel personally 'safe' because of the availability of healthcare free at point of use, but also happy that that safety extends to others in society. Lee Ridley, a comedian with cerebral palsy, goes further, pointing out the lottery of circumstances which can make healthcare vital: "But the fact that I'm still here to tell the tale says everything you need to know about how vital it is. Not just for people like myself, but for everyone. Because let's face it, you'll never know when you'll need the help of the NHS until it happens" (Lee Ridley).

Our third theme – the NHS as a source of pride in Britain – is complex but highly significant across the campaigns. The NHS is described as beloved because of what it does for British society: "It is magic. But it's a magic that was created consciously by people who were thinking about society and thinking about others. It's a magic that grows out of a certain kind of social unselfishness" (Brian Eno). Eno's assertion of what we can be proud of about the NHS focuses on the 'unselfishness' that he perceives in its creation. Also foregrounding the NHS's history, multiple videos emphasise the intergenerational transmission of this care: 'Our families have built this service' (Charlotte Church); 'it was there to support my parents, my grandparents it's been there to support my children and my grandchildren' (Dave Ward); 'save our NHS for ourselves and for future generations' (Margaret Greenwood). These statements celebrate the NHS as an inheritance from past generations to pass on, safely, to future generations.

These contributions identify the NHS as a locus of national unity, both retrospective and prospective, over the decades. This asserts that the putative *sacrifices* entailed by the risk-pooling of a universal tax-funded system, are justified by those of prior generations, and generations yet to come. In so doing they also invoke what Fitzgerald et al (2020) critique as a problematic 'politics of heredity': the implicit and, occasionally, explicit sense that entitlements to NHS care are a question of 'inherited entitlements' rather than a right to care for those currently resident in the UK. There are campaign contributions which resist the nativist basis of such generational claims: as Shami Chakrabarti's video puts it, acknowledging the imperial staffing of the early NHS: 'It's our national treasure but it was built by people from all over the world.' Nonetheless, a vision of the NHS as affectively powerful because of its cross-generational role, can easily elide into anti-migrant discourses, nativism and welfare chauvinism (Ketola and Nordensvard, 2018; Speed and Mannion, 2020).

Beyond these references to generational care, other segments of these campaigns propose an alternative, and more expansive focus on society as 'everyone that we share this country with':

'Because it's a national kindness that we all contribute together to make sure everyone is cared for. No matter who they are, everyone gets looked after. It's a national selflessness.' (David Tennant)

'A safety net um for yourself and for your friends and family but also just for everyone you pass on the street. Everywhere, everyone that we share this country with.' (Jonathan Ross)

'That's what's so wonderful about the NHS. It's an act of love, it's what society gives to itself to look after everybody in that society.' (Michael Rosen)

It is, of course, a comfortable self-identity to live in a society that one can suggest is marked by 'unselfishness', 'kindness' and 'love'. For those suspicious of nationalistic tropes, the NHS holds out the comfort of solidarity, without the more jingiostic connotations of the nation. Multiple videos and campaign pages credit as making them feel not just glad to have the NHS but *proud* to be British.

'The National Health Service is the most civilized thing about Britain.' (Jeremy Corbyn)

'I believe it's our country's finest social achievement.' (Margaret Greenwood)

'The NHS is probably the thing that makes me proudest to be British.' (David Tennant)

'There's so much talk about patriotism right now but there's nothing more red, white and blue than the blue and white of the NHS.' (Shami Chakrabarti)

Charlotte Church's video ends: 'What would we be without [the NHS]'. I went back and checked the transcript here, in case the transcription software had misunderstood her Welsh accent and she had said "where would we be without it"; a more commonplace assertion of the need for medical care and a societal safety net. But no, she twice says *what* would we be, and the phrase has stayed with me since. These videos demonstrate the extent to which loving the NHS can become an identity and not merely an opinion or sentiment to be held. For left-wing campaigners seeking shared ground in a divided country post-Brexit, post-empire and post-COVID (Stanley, 2022), the NHS is a unifying affiliation.

Saving the NHS, one hospital at a time

Local campaigns against service reconfigurations and hospital downgrades and closures are distinct from but heavily nested within broader campaigning around protecting 'the NHS'. Photographs of communities resisting hospital closure, with placards, at protest events, and via petitions, are a longstanding image associated with UK health politics. As I've suggested with co-authors elsewhere (Stewart, 2019; Dodworth and Stewart, 2022; Stewart, Dodworth and Ercia, 2022), public practices of campaigning have often been referred to, but rarely studied within empirical research on the organisation of healthcare in the UK. Where empirical research on members of the UK responding to hospital closures *has* taken place, understanding the perspectives of campaigners is rarely the focus. Much contemporary scholarship has departed from, and thus perpetuated, a policy-driven account of public responses to hospital closures. Sometimes the inclusion of one or two public interviewees within a wider cohort of staff interviews simply adds weight to staff perceptions of public views (Fulop et al, 2012). The use of discrete choice experiments, where public interviewees are funnelled into organisationally-defined tradeoffs (such as between patient safety and travel time to hospitals) (Barratt et al, 2015), and their responses to these dilemmas measured, epitomises the analytic dilemmas of a policy-framed approach. This approach lacks sensitivity to context and openness to exploring research participants' own sense-making (Jones, Fraser and Stewart, 2019). As others have concluded (Dalton et al, 2016; Djellouli et al, 2019), the top-down focus of most studies means that we know relatively little, in academic terms, about public opposition to hospital closures in the NHS. In this section, I report on how hospital campaigners describe their campaigning work, focusing on the connections they describe between their local campaigns and the national NHS, and on the tactics they employ to try to protect local hospitals.

When describing the value of the local hospitals they sought to defend, campaigners often referenced the NHS as a marker of quality, in the context of their descriptions of the ways in which their own local experience was high quality: 'The whole point of this NHS is to serve the people, you know, that's what it was set up for to provide care, the best care possible' (CSO.CS3.P1). Similarly to the national campaigns discussed, references to the best care were rarely defined with reference to cutting-edge technology or clinical techniques. Clinical justifications for many of the closures studied were about how technology reduced the need for bed capacity with quicker recovery times. Accordingly, as argued elsewhere (Stewart, 2019), threatened hospitals tended to be valued for their delivery of familiar person-centred care, predicated on caring relationships between staff (often known to patients) and patients.

In several of the campaigns studied, the reconfiguration of services meant that local hospitals were defined as 'options' to be appraised as alternative sites for delivery of care. Thus local hospitals, and the communities campaigning to save them, were essentially in competition with each other. However, often to the frustration of managers faced with defined budgets, campaigners tended to resist these tradeoffs: "We want to help to protect our whole health economy, not just our hospital, you know, public health, our health visitors, our school nurses etc, we also need to protect those services" (Linda, female campaigner, HF.E).

Far from accepting what managers and politicians argued was the necessity of making 'tough decisions' within a fixed budget envelope, campaigners more often presented saving their one hospital as a means to a broader effort to save the NHS as a whole. In one interview, a campaigner explicitly linked their short-term aim of saving services at one hospital, to a grander project to reform the governance of healthcare in Northern Ireland towards greater community voice:

'The shorter term aim would be to stop the Trust and the Department of Health from taking away services – acute services – from the Hospital and centralising them. So that was the second aim, the shorter term aim. And the other aim I suppose longer term too ... but short term as well would be to reform the NHS governance, how the NHS here is governed in terms of its management, to radically reform that. Now those are very big aims to have and very ambitious aims, but the group was established to give the community some voice or campaigning voice outside of local council government structures to try and campaign for those aims.' (Jeffrey, male campaigner, HF.NI)

In this way, local campaigns were linked to national efforts. Rather than accepting the premise of local managers that centralisation was how to save the NHS, campaigners across multiple different hospitals saw local engagement, and the protection of services, as a way forward for the wider NHS (Stewart, Dodworth and Erica, 2022).

As the campaigns we studied progressed, relations between NHS decision-makers and community campaigns often became increasingly oppositional. Communication breakdowns and a lack of transparency were experienced as not merely problematic parts of an engagement process, but as unacceptable in the context of a state-owned national service: "I'm not sure where the decision was finally made. I don't know who finally made it. ... And that's wrong, I think, you should know, I think. 'Cause you're paying into this National Health Service, so you own it. And as an owner and a user, you should know" (Sam, female campaigner, CSO.CS4).

Reflecting Cowan's (2020) discussion of campaigners becoming suspicious about the opacity of contemporary NHS processes, frustrations about transparency often tipped over into a belief that managers were deliberately seeking to evade scrutiny or input from communities:

'We believe that there is a plan, when I say we, we healthcare activists, believe there is a plan, it's not just a belief, you know, there's a clear plan of closing vital local services in particular our DGHs [District General Hospitals] and our maternities in order to save money.' (James, male campaigner, CSO.CS3)

In this case, the interviewee's immediate concern about the removal of a particular set of services in his local community had developed into a much broader frustration at a perceived absence of democratic control over what were seen as collective assets.

In interviews, some campaigners de-emphasised the clinical roles hospitals play in favour of a broader project of strengthening local community facilities, especially in contexts of actual or perceived decline:

'When you took anything out of a local community, a Post Office or a local hospital, it's ... you're taking part of the heart away from that community. And ... like, if we were trying to attract more investment ... one of the key arguments we'd use to attract investment ... would be that you have a local acute hospital to service your staff if you want to come here.' (Jeffrey, male campaigner, HF.NI)

'I don't see a hospital just as a building in its entirety, it's everything that goes on in a hospital and so I felt that the post office it relocating ... and, you know, it's going down to a wee shop. I don't want to sound disparaging but, you know, you would pass that and never give it a blink, but the post office had a presence. The hospital's got a presence and even the recycling place – at least there's something on a Saturday and Sunday, a place of social interaction because it's not open during the week so people go down there. I actually felt that, you know, it was creating a ... for me, and I am using the word bereavement, but this is going to cause a real bereavement.' (Elsie, female campaigner, CSO.CS1)

Social interaction, evidence of a community's resilience to attract external employers, the 'heart' of a community: these aspects of a hospital campaign demonstrate the weight of expectation resting on NHS facilities, especially in non-urban areas where other amenities are more scarce (Stewart, 2019). NHS facilities in this framing are cast as an anchor institution, similar to, but *more* important than, any other public service.

In one community hospital closure in rural Scotland, two lead campaigners assumed an institutionally-versed approach to their advocacy, leveraging legal, policy and local politics instruments at different levels of the system to combat what local NHS managers. Experiential knowledge of the hospital and its model of care was less prominent in their strategy. The lead campaigner reiterated that: "This isn't about NHS and so on, but it's about democracy and the changes to democracy ... I suggest throughout the whole of the bloody [region] – how do they wish to promote and process democracy?" (David, male campaigner, CSO.CS1).

These campaigners primarily directed their opposition to the local management of the 'NHS' itself. This seemingly encompassed the board and clinical staff but also perceived faceless bureaucrats and managers making, on their account, unaccountable and non-transparent decisions. Part of the campaigners' efforts, therefore, was to reinsert 'politics' into decisions that had been deliberately depoliticised through bureaucratic process and anonymity:

'[W]hen I have emails back from NHS [Region] and so on, you ask them some questions "we won't talk about that because it's politics"; the whole thing is bloody politics, you can't divide the things through ... so you know, for me that's a lame duck excuse to get out of answering difficult questions.' (David, male campaigner, CSO.CS1)

For this campaign, the NHS was symptomatic of a growing democratic deficit in British institutions but also of a now entrenched managerialism. This monolithic portrayal of the NHS bureaucracy as threat to local culture was unusual among our cases.

In another, highly politicised proposed closure, campaigners instead described themselves as deeply embedded within local networks of NHS expertise, clinical knowledge and above all *values* in opposition to 'the government' of the day. They emphasised the strength and objectivity of 'their' clinicians' arguments in shared response to the proposed changes – the epitome of credentialled knowledge:

'First of all we did our own critique of the proposal. ... So I think the first people to start writing about it were the A&E doctors and they just wrote an analysis, they critiqued the proposal was full of false ... rubbish, evidence was wrong, percentages that were wrong, facts that were just demonstrably wrong; so they did that and then I think the ITU Intensive Therapy Unit people did that and they talked about training, the impact on training etc., and then the maternity people and then we had public health did it and ... then we got contributions from GP practices, about five or six practices wrote, and then we wrote as trainers because it would've destroyed GP training [locally] because they actually use the hospital. So we had lots of very, very high level ... these are frontline professionals who are clever and know their stuff and got together and did rounded critiques.' (Linda, female campaigner, HF.E)

This evidence, and the judicial review it informed, was in this campaign about 'reclaiming power' (Linda) from national politics, resonating with what Newman (2012) describes as antagonistic knowledge work. This closely resembled the words of a campaigner from a different hospital, who reiterated:

'[W]e realised from an early stage that ... the clinical arguments that would ... have the most force in all this. ... [M]any politicians and many senior bureaucrats would argue, "the evidence states this", but they don't actually produce the evidence. So you're living in a, sort of, post-truth society in that sense, where you've always now got to ask for the evidence all of the time. And we didn't see much evidence. In fact our evidence showed the opposite.' (Jeffrey, male campaigner, HF.NI)

Here, credentialled sources of knowledge produced by experts *within* the NHS not only have weight, but provide the final bastion against politically driven assaults on knowledge, 'truth' and evidence production. At the same time, such strongly credentialed knowledge was democratised and given meaning by its experiential 'connection' to the people, to whom the NHS 'belongs' (Linda). Through this epistemic labour, clinical and public campaigners re-inscribed the NHS as both an authoritative and public institution.

Questions of ownership of local facilities also loomed large in other cases, especially where the hospitals under threat were small community facilities. In one such case, campaigners again emphasised the (pre-NHS) history of their hospital, funded as a community war memorial in the aftermath of World War One. In this quote, the campaigner highlights how the history of the hospital, at the heart of the community, was inscribed and re-inscribed by cultural rituals of remembering:

'There's lots of really nice stories about how the money was collected; some of them involving somebody going on a bike round all the neighbouring villages actually physically collecting the money, so there was one main sort of benefactor and the boards are, you know, there's the inscriptions are all there down at the hospital, so it is a war memorial hospital. So there's that sense of history there, you know, every year the remembrance service, normally they would be at public sort of open spaces whereas at [here] it's actually in the hospital so, you know, people troop round from the church and then they lay the wreath actually in the hospital.' (Karen, female campaigner, CSO.CS2)

This emphasises that, as Gosling (2017) has noted, the 1948 creation of the NHS is merely one event in the histories of older former voluntary hospitals within their communities.

Campaigners often argued that these longstanding relationships created a responsibility on local NHS managers to engage effectively with local communities about change.

'Everyone thought they [NHS managers] were lying because patently their actions were different to what they were saying, and also they wouldn't answer at a level that the public could understand and I think that's a fault of the NHS everywhere and I have to constantly remind myself not to get caught up in this institutional speak.' (Robert, male campaigner, HF.W)

This (one-time) campaigner had advocated successfully for new, credible evidence generation (in collaboration with a local university) on models of delivering rural services. He saw re-establishing public trust as a crucial part of that: 'Part of the evidence base needs to be the sort of contract between the people and the deliverers.' In the face of longstanding mistrust of healthcare reconfiguration over time, the importance and symbolism of retaining and defending local hospitals became a proxy for fears over broader reductions in service:

'It appears to me that all the power in the NHS is in the secondary care and in the public's mind at the moment the most important thing as far as healthcare delivery is a hospital, and actually until the NHS can demonstrate you don't have to walk through a hospital door to get these services, that's what the public get and you can't blame them, you know, they want to know they're safe.' (Robert, male campaigner, HEW)

Conclusion

Reflecting on changes on tactics across the decades, Crane (2019) argues that 'NHS activism has been made and remade over time, following the conscious efforts of campaigners'. The 'repertoires of contention' (Della Porta, 2013) I describe in this chapter are recursive – in that publics draw inspiration from related campaigns – but not static, in that they innovate and respond to changing contexts. This chapter has reported some of the complex work that sits around, shapes and feeds off photogenic moments of protests in contemporary hospital campaigns (Dodworth and Stewart, 2022; see also Stewart, Dodworth and Erica, 2022). This includes strategic decisions about when and how to organise visible public protests, as an alternative or supplement to 'behind the scenes' influencing, 'knowledge work' (Newman, 2012) or 'information-based campaigning' (Crane, 2019). By contrast, my analysis of national campaigns explores the visible end products of extensive invisible labour: no doubt the casual celebrity videos I analyse were the outcome of many meetings, decisions and, indeed, social networks.

My concern is for what campaigns might tell us about how Britain loves the NHS now, exploring campaigning in order to better understand the peculiar contemporary relationship between British publics and their healthcare system. While public mobilisations are a significant trend in health politics globally (Geiger, 2021), NHS campaigning has an unusually conservative character: what stands out from examining these local and national campaigns is their essentially preservationist goals. The vision of campaigning for the NHS presented in this chapter is one that is not grounded in reform. Indeed in recent years scholars have repeatedly suggested that we *cannot* successfully reform the NHS from within a frame of public 'love' for it (Cowan, 2020; Arnold-Forster and Gainty, 2021). Rather, the campaigns described here are at root seeking to protect and restore a vision of the NHS 'as intended'. In her ethnographic research on activism in the NHS, Cowan (2020) repeatedly references nostalgia for a 1950s model of healthcare as core component of campaigning for the NHS. While the national campaigns analysed here exhibit nostalgia, certainly, they are also underpinned by a more substantive commitment to the NHS as a set of principles; a sturdy, reliable safety net for all who 'share this country'. Campaign webpages were clear that migrant charges, for example, were 'an attack on our communities and the basic principles of the NHS'. Threats to the NHS, especially from the looming spectre of 'American healthcare' (Lorne, 2022) (understood in campaign materials not only as terrifying alternative reality but as an active threat already stealthily 'embedded' into our system), prompt a battle mentality that is energising, if not always illuminating. Local hospital campaigns are also explicitly seeking to prevent proposed changes to services, and those studied rarely presented a novel vision of healthcare locally, more often appealing to the familiarity of how services recently operated.

From an international perspective it is also notable that the NHS campaigning explored in this chapter is rarely explicitly consumeristic. Campaigners' demands are almost never couched in terms of individual needs or preferences. In both local and national campaigning we see the interplay of mobilisations of patient experience with more formal, population-level arguments that mimic the 'official' credentialed knowledge of the state (Rabeharisoa, Moreira and Akrich, 2014; Stewart, Dodworth and Erica, 2022). This can be understood as an implicit message of the recurrent 'our NHS' narrative: not a consumeristic demand for service but an assertion of the system as a collective endeavour between population, professions and state. Local campaigns also act to decentre the notion of the NHS as singular institution located only or primarily within the political-administrative bodies of the state: asserting a stake in healthcare as a coproduction between state, professionals, and communities (Stewart, 2021). Writing a decade into the New Labour era, Newman and Clarke argue that the 'citizen-consumer binary' lacks traction with public views about healthcare in the UK. Reflecting on people's preferences about being called citizen, consumer, patient or service user, they suggest that these are 'identifications, rather than identities: they are about imagined or desired forms of attachment and belonging to domains, institutions, practices and people' (Clarke and Newman, 2007, p 754). This chapter investigates the way that people articulate and mobilise their imagined and desired visions of the NHS through the work of campaigning.

6

Using and loving the NHS

The previous chapters have sought to demonstrate the range of ways in which members of the British public interact with the NHS, shedding greater light on how donating time and money, and campaigning to protect or 'save' the NHS are important facets of societal engagement. In this chapter, I explore how the context of societal care for the NHS shapes experiences of service use. It is not always customary to understand the way patients use services a mode of participation in our healthcare system: it is often seen as private, and not public action. In a previous book (Stewart, 2016), I argued that separating out accounts of service use from accounts of citizen participation neglects the ways in which service use constitutes creative and tactical action, and risks missing out how swathes of the population exercise agency in healthcare, not through formalised 'choice' but by 'playing the system' to achieve an acceptable outcome. Several respected and valued colleagues told me that this was a step too far, over-extending the definition of participation and straying unhelpfully beyond disciplinary boundaries. This invokes a putative distinction between sociological study of people's (private) experiences of healthcare, and political science or public policy study of how healthcare is organised and managed.

The consistent suggestion that not only *can* we separate out our roles as patient, and as citizen, within a health system, but that for analytic clarity we *should* do so, continues to strike me as misguided. In this chapter I present an analysis of how and when people providing online reviews of care received in the UK NHS talk about the NHS. Others have explored the way in which patient experience has come to be instrumentalised within healthcare systems and used as not just a barometer of quality of healthcare but as a mechanism for financial incentives within the system (Edwards, Staniszewska and Crichton, 2004; Montgomery et al, 2022). Existing research suggests that providing these online reviews – which a minority of patients do – has a specific function around caring for care:

> Interviewees provided feedback because they cared about the NHS as a national resource, which, *as citizens*, they felt a sense of responsibility for. At the same time, many interviewees or their family members were receiving care from specific services and professionals. Thus, *as patients*, they had to navigate the power inequalities, vulnerabilities and dependencies implicit in care relations (Martin et al, 2015). These

two dimensions – *caring for* the NHS as a symbolic entity invested with emotional and ethical weight, whilst being dependent on *care from* NHS services and healthcare professionals – provides essential background for contextualising the practices of people providing online feedback about public healthcare services in the UK. (Mazanderani et al, 2021, p 5)

This analysis helpfully distinguishes the provision of feedback from a consumeristic act: acknowledging the complex and often hybrid roles that patients have within an NHS system (Clarke et al, 2007).

My determination to include a chapter on service use within this book on how Britain loves the NHS rests on two interlinked claims. One is empirical: I will argue that the way we feel and talk about actual experiences of healthcare in the UK is strongly filtered through the way we feel and talk about 'the NHS' as 'symbolic entity invested with emotional and ethical weight' (Mazanderani et al, 2021). The analysis that follows identifies recurring references to the NHS which, I suggest, support that claim. This makes large-scale comparisons of healthcare experience across different health systems – disentangling how members of the public feel about their own experiences of healthcare, current approaches to organising healthcare, and the institutional context of the healthcare system – extremely challenging (Larsen, 2020; Burlacu and Roescu, 2021).

The stronger claim is a normative one about how we *should* research and know healthcare. There is no lack of research published about people's experiences of particular forms of care (Edwards, Staniszewska and Crichton, 2004). Especially within the sub-discipline of sociology of health and illness this work goes beyond Likert scale quantifications of patient satisfaction towards qualitative studies which are rich with meaning, exploring not merely whether healthcare 'works' (achieving its clinically-defined goals) but what difference it makes to the individual wellbeing and self-image of patients. This research does, though, intersect only lightly with research on the policy and organisation of healthcare systems. As General Practitioner and author Gavin Francis puts it: 'Hospital is a place dedicated to the efficient processing of thousands of people; the hopes and anxieties of individuals tend to get drowned out in the crowd" (Francis, 2015). There are of course exceptions in both healthcare practice and research: Edwards, Staniszewska and Crichton (2004) explicitly centre the question of whether and how patient reports of their experiences might be used as a barometer of quality of care. By contrast, when reading key accounts of the NHS as a healthcare system, and especially its historiography, the actual bodily, material, joyful and tragic interactions which constitute healthcare recede, in favour of viewpoints grounded in the experience, concerns and priorities of politicians, clinicians and managers.

My suggestion is both that sociology of health and illness requires more consistent engagement with the organisation and financing of healthcare (a point already made by sociologists such as Davies, 2003), and that studies of healthcare organisation and health systems needs to engage more consistently with intimate and embodied experiences of patients as the crux of what is particular about the business of healthcare. As scholars, we need to find a register to discuss healthcare which neither neglects the critical, often life-altering significance of *patient* perspectives on a health system, nor delegitimises a broader perspective in which citizens might assess the merits of a particular system. Particularly in an NHS system where governmental responsibility for health security is broadly accepted, these standpoints are integrated in most people's daily lives. When I attend hospital for an appointment, or navigate to the NHS website to assuage my worries about a poorly child, I do so as both patient and a member of society, aware that my service use is nested within a broader system of resources and priorities. Placing patient experiences of care at the centre of healthcare system research rejects the suggestion that we encounter the health system as either patient (with all its attendant vulnerabilities) or citizen (with all its association of power and agency), and foregrounds how we integrate both (Clarke et al, 2007).

Care Opinion as a platform for feedback

Formal structures have existed since the 1970s to offer some representation of patients and the public within health service decision-making (Newbigging, 2016 offers a helpful review). As well as varying over time, reflecting contemporaneous visions of what 'good' public and patient involvement might look like, these structures have differed in England, Northern Ireland, Scotland and Wales. Given these differences, there is no single organisation which represents patient and public views about the NHS across the UK. In this chapter, I rely instead on Care Opinion, a UK-wide platform for patient reviews, which has the added advantage of offering relatively unfiltered narratives of healthcare service use.

Practices of online reviewing of everything from restaurants to films to businesses are deeply entrenched into contemporary social life. They are also increasingly part of the context of health systems (Montgomery et al, 2022). Care Opinion is an online platform where members of the public can submit 'stories' of up to 1000 words, linking them to the different 'provider' organisations they interacted with during their care. Created in 2005, it was initially seen as part of the expansion of patient choice within the NHS in England (Appleby, Harrison and Devlin, 2003) but its role has evolved into a focus on collaborative quality improvement: as its founder described 'turn[ing] the moving, thoughtful and reflective stories that people share into better health and social care services' (Hodgkin, 2013). As a non-profit-making Community Interest Company, Care Opinion's business model is to sell subscriptions to health and social care organisations who can make use of the patient stories. In England these subscriptions are from specific provider organisations, but in Scotland and in Northern Ireland, Care Opinion has been contracted by the Scottish Government and Public Health Agency respectively (Care Opinion, 2022a). While Care Opinion therefore shares some similarities with private digital platforms which Lupton (2014) argues have commodified patient experience (see also Mazanderani and Powell, 2013), this is a non-profit-making platform which, through these contractual arrangements with NHS organisations, has become interwoven with the NHS. The idea of Care Opinion as a useful broker between patient experience and organisational improvement has been supported by research which has found that staff value the learning (Baines et al, 2021) and that reviews might capture safety incidents which have otherwise gone unreported through official channels (Gillespie and Reader, n.d.). The decision to submit a Care Opinion review is a voluntary one on the part of the service user. Patients are, though, encouraged to do so by subscriber organisations within the NHS, for example via posters and leaflets in waiting areas, so they can reply to stories directly.

My search filter aimed to capture reviews which did not simply describe an experience of care (whether negative or positive) but which specifically discussed the 'NHS' within the body text of the narrative. In order to create a manageable corpus, I searched only for stories tagged as being about emergency medicine. This specialism was chosen because it is one of the main 'front doors' to NHS care, and also because it is often a particularly visible pressure point in the broader healthcare system, especially given very public waiting time targets (Iacobucci, 2019; Thorlby, Gardner and Turton, 2019). However it also has other characteristics likely to change the way people express feedback: people are more likely than in other specialisms to have one-off experiences with an emergency department, and the process of triage is particularly uncertain, especially with heightened 'right care' campaigns about appropriate service use. I discuss how these dimensions of emergency care might influence the analysis later in the chapter. I applied text searching for any stories with 'NHS' in the body of the story, and manually removed stories where the reference was to, for example, a specific organisation (for example, NHS Lothian) rather than the NHS as a more general entity. This left 197 stories from 2019 (out of a total number of 352 emergency medicine stories) and 221 stories from 2021 (out of a total number of 634 emergency medicine stories).

Care Opinion does not collect reliable demographic data about stories, but one option to contextualise the nature of this corpus of stories, and its relationship to the broader body of patient stories, is to explore the criticality rating applied to each. Care Opinion moderators (that is, Care Opinion staff, rather than NHS staff) assign a criticality rating to each story shared,

Table 6.1: Proportions of Care Opinion stories scored as having no critical comment

	2019	2021
Emergency medicine stories with standalone mention of 'NHS'	72% no critical comment	63% no critical comment
All emergency medicine stories	70% no critical comment	57% no critical comment

from 0 (not critical) to 5 (very critical) on the basis of reported emotional or physical harm to the patient in the story (Berry et al, 2022). Berry et al (2022) describe the role of moderators more fully and discuss the process of scoring. It is important to note that Care Opinion data cannot be used as a straightforward measure of the quality of patient care across the country. Highly critical stories are likely not to be submitted on Care Opinion (Berry et al, 2022), perhaps because anonymous feedback is not 'actionable', and formal complaints processes might be preferred (Locock et al, 2020; Speed, Davison and Gunnell, 2016). Additionally, there is longstanding evidence that patients may reinterpret their experiences in a positive light (Edwards, Staniszewska and Crichton, 2004). However, Table 6.1 offers two useful insights.

First, it shows that stories making standalone mention of 'the' or 'our NHS' are marginally less critical overall then the broader body of stories. Second, it shows a shift over time period: emergency medicine stories in 2021 were more critical than those submitted in 2019.

Understanding patient stories as NHS stories

Analysing hundreds of stories is a peculiar and emotional experience. While some are general and brief, many stories are highly affecting, containing personal details and fleeting mentions of moments of joy, relief, devastation and loss. Acknowledging this, Berry et al's (2022) ethnographic research with Care Opinion moderators reports staff sharing positive stories between them to lighten the load of the more harrowing tales. The work of reading and coding them as a researcher can feel intrusive, even though consent for reuse for research is built into the platform (Munro, 2015). I returned often to Shapiro's (2011) call for us to balance critical inquiry with 'narrative humility' when dealing with the stories patients choose to tell. Despite the very wide range of different conditions and services described, stories also, over time, begin to display repetitive elements. Sometimes this is about what is described; for example the recurrent weight attached to a timely cup of tea as a symbol of care. As a perplexed German colleague put it to me, on analysing social media data on a different project, 'what is it with this country and tea?' More often it is about elements of narrative structure; recurrences in the way that stories begin, progress, and end. Through the thematic analysis I identified recurrent elements of how people's described experiences of care were discursively connected to 'the NHS', and the ways in which this seemed to encourage particular descriptions of self and of organisational encounters.

A credit to the NHS

One feature of this analysis that surprised me was the relatively high number of very short stories, comprising only a few sentences, and often lacking much detail. The overwhelming purpose of such stories was not to communicate substantive, let alone actionable, feedback on details of care received but to express gratitude. The following is the whole story submitted by one patient: "I was recently in hospital at [location]. I cannot compliment the staff of A&E and Ward 2 enough. All were so kind and caring – real credits to our NHS!" (story from 2019, criticality rating 0).

As this example demonstrates, short and positive stories are often effusive, including exclamation marks. Descriptions of care are often accompanied by descriptions of staff as 'angels' or 'real life superheroes'. Relatedly, in the absence of conventional signoffs (given the anonymity of the platform) many stories end with brief stock phrases, sometimes using a heart or thankyou emoticon: 'Our wonderful NHS', 'proud of the NHS', 'keep up the good work!' These can be understood as the 'coda' (Labov, 1997) of the story: it signals the end of a narrative and, as Labov (1997) puts it 'puts *off* a question' by ending on a positive note.

From a consumeristic perspective – in which feedback is given either to 'voice' an objection or to offer ammunition for other consumers to choose to 'exit' a failing provider (Needham, 2009) – such stories are bewildering. Even acknowledging that people are often short of time, the lack of substantive content makes the decision to offer a written review seem perplexing. However from the position of both invested stakeholder, and indeed a scared or suffering human grateful for human connection in a vulnerable moment, the prevalence of grateful, and somehow insubstantial stories makes much more sense. Mazanderani et al identified this in their interviews about online feedback:

> Feedback practices were shaped by *both* their embodied experiences of care (good and bad) *and* a strong moral commitment to, indeed a sense of responsibility toward, other patients and service users, healthcare professionals and services, as well as 'the NHS' as a highly symbolic national resource. (Mazanderani et al, 2021, p 6)

Many stories seem intended to find a public expression of gratitude, and as Mazanderani et al's interviewees suggest, this was often explicitly in a context where the NHS was felt to be 'knocked' in public discourse. One interviewee in that study remarked: "I think doctors and nurses need to hear that we're grateful and not just turn on the TV and see the NHS is crumbling around our knees" (female, 36). In this context, the recurrent codas – grateful expressions of thanks such as 'thankyou NHS' – function to leave the reader with an overall sense of things having gone well. In their analysis of patient comments on the NHS Choices website, Brookes et al (2022) suggest that codas to positive stories are intended for both other patients and for providers themselves to read, while codas to negative stories have a more restricted imagined audience of other patients. In grateful stories, the connection between the attribution of credit to individuals *and* to the entire healthcare system can be difficult to understand: "All in all we cannot thank the NHS enough for their excellent service, especially a great big thank you to Angela for calming us down and assuring us everything was fine" (story from 2021, criticality rating 0). The elision between 'the NHS' and the many staff who work within it is a familiar one from broader cultural representation of healthcare in the UK (Saunders, 2022). Note, for example, how Michael Rosen's bestselling book about his experiences of healthcare during a life-threatening experience of COVID-19, filled with remarkably poignant letters from health professionals who cared for him, is "a story of life, death and the NHS" (Rosen, 2021).

Even in longer, more substantial stories, gratitude is very often the overall focus. The very common phrase 'a credit to the NHS' is frequently used to praise individual or groups of staff. 'All the staff were outstanding but Maria was the pinnacle of what makes the NHS fabulous, Thank you!' (story from 2019, criticality rating 0). This is interesting both in that 'the NHS' becomes not the experience being discussed but the yardstick or standard by which that experience might be measured. Furthermore, as in this story, the compliment of being a 'credit to' or even 'the pinnacle' of the NHS appears overwhelmingly to be attributed to acts of kindness and caring, rather than in reference to clinical aspects of care. Stories analysed were relatively quiet about clinical aspects of care received, let alone references to technology or sophisticated pathways. Likely reflecting a focus on thanking staff, stories are much more often focused on human aspects of care. These include holding a patient's hand when they receive bad news ("held his hand when he was told about his brain tumour and reassured him. He told us he had a wee 'greet' since he knew the seriousness of it" [story from 2021, criticality rating 0]); using humour to lighten difficult moments ("everyone was amazing they even managed to get me laughing and totally took my mind off the situation" [story from 2019, criticality rating 0]); and careful reassurance ("she listened to me and reassured me in my panicked state that everything was going to be ok" [story from 2019, criticality rating 0]). The intersection of care and vulnerability here is a powerful one: "I would like to say how wonderful each and every member of the team who I met were. They were caring, compassionate and professional and made me feel safe during a very overwhelming scary experience, where I felt at my most vulnerable" (story from 2021, criticality rating 0). As this excerpt suggests, critical moments in the narratives often combine a moment of (sometimes life-threatening) vulnerability and uncertainty for the patient; and the ability of a team of health professionals to temper the associated fear.

The presentation of self in scene-setting

Longer stories often display the classical structural components of narrative including abstract (summary), orientation in time and place, complicating action, evaluation, resolution and coda (Labov, 1997; Riessman, 2008). Many longer and more substantial patient stories begin with an orienting scene-setting paragraph, in which the writer explains where and when the care occurred. This is, at least in Labov's view, a universal element of narrative structure. Distinctively though, in the pressured emergency medicine context of these narratives, the scene setting is also significantly focused on a favourable 'presentation of self'. That is, writers provided details to reassure the imagined reader that they, or (if submitting a story of another person's care) the patient in question, is legitimate, virtuous, or unusually vulnerable.

Efforts to present the visit to Accident & Emergency as appropriate drew on a number of different sources of legitimacy. Commonly, narratives refer to being instructed to seek emergency care by someone with medical knowledge or authority. Sometimes this is a phone call to either 999, a GP, or NHS 111, for example: "Have had to go to A&E three times within the last few days, due to covid complications. It was not my decision to go – I was taken twice by emergency ambulance and the other time, when no ambulances were available, by car" (story from 2021, criticality rating 3).

In another story, a patient describes the emotional toll of identifying the most appropriate route to care, contrasting her GP receptionist with a triage nurse:

'The receptionist at my GP's was very kind and concerned. This helped as I was scared. At A&E when I was triaged the nurse said "you'll be here for hours you could still make your GP or pharmacist". I asked if she thought I should go home, that this wasn't serious. I also told her the GP advised me to come. I felt quite tearful and worried I was wasting NHS time.' (Story from 2021, criticality rating 2)

Navigating routes into emergency care often seemed both difficult and worrying in people's accounts of care. Patient stories often suggested that arriving at the hospital by ambulance (following a 999 call) was the most legitimate route to attending A&E, with triage by a paramedic providing reassurance of clinical need. "I appreciate you've got to be fairly tough to work in A&E, but to be shouted at by a doctor because you 'shouldn't be here' (it was 999 who took me there, but never mind), & belittled for having medical conditions they hadn't heard of" (story from 2021, criticality rating 3).

NHS 111 and informal referrals from primary care, by contrast, are a less reliable arbiter, in that many narratives recount taking advice to go to Accident & Emergency and there being treated as *illegitimate*:

'The nurse asked me why I was in ED this evening. I attempted to answer the question but failed to do so as the nurse spoke over me every time and said "there's nothing we can do for you here this evening you have a long term condition"! I advised her I knew that as did my GP who sent me to ED following a discussion with a Dr at the hospital.' (Story from 2021, criticality rating 2)

Here, the spectre of timewasting (being a timewaster, being seen or treated as a timewaster, and, crucially, feeling reassured that everyone knows one is *not* a timewaster once triage has taken place) played a major role (Llanwarne et al, 2017):

'Felt really nervous, and I hated that an ambulance had to come as I never like to pull on resources from the NHS as they're so busy.' (Story from 2021, criticality rating 0)

'I came home and burst into tears feeling deflated and upset. I felt I was a burden on the NHS as it was a weekend, no beds and COVID and I would just have to await my turn.' (Story from 2021, criticality rating 3)

People who had attended Accident & Emergency in the absence of an ambulance or formal medical advice often referred to broader structures of credentialed medical knowledge: a family member or colleague who was a health professional and who advised them to get urgent care.

Across the whole corpus of patient stories, examples of feeling that concerns had *not* been taken seriously, are common. In some cases such stories include a description of a 'victory' of the patient's need for medical care having been proved legitimate after triage, sometimes with grim predictions for what might have happened if the patient had not persevered. These are, in common with earlier excerpts, depicted not only as a *private* medical experience but as a *public* claim on medical help. One unusual example makes a formally-worded apology for using emergency care with*out* a 'legitimate' reason:

'I would like to apologise for having accessed A and E for what turned out to be a sprained ankle as I am aware this could have been dealt with elsewhere but I greatly appreciate the time and care taken by all staff to reassure me that this was not something more serious and to provide advice personal to me and my situation.' (Story from 2019, criticality rating 1)

In contrast to stories of brusque or dismissive care for problems seen as illegitimate, this story expresses appreciation for staff providing reassurance and person-centred advice. The framing of the story is both grateful for kindness and advice received but fundamentally apologetic for having made what is perceived as an unnecessary request on this most pressured gateway to NHS care.

This overt apology relates to another facet of how story writers present themselves (sometimes co-existing with, and sometimes substituting for legitimacy); virtue. Here, descriptions of self focus not only on the described visit as a legitimate one, but on how *little* they ask from the NHS in general: "Was at A&E today, having been fortunate enough to have never needed a trip to hospital for last 20 years or so" (story from 2019, criticality rating 0), and: "Not having the requirement to attend A&E or a Hospital since I cannot remember when" (story from 2019, criticality rating 0).

Some of these go further, interweaving accounts of good fortune with aspects of their lifestyle that have reduced their healthcare needs: "I am back to my normal very active life, for which I will always be eternally grateful. I have been lucky and needed very little help from the NHS throughout my life" (story from 2021, criticality rating 0).

In one long and complex narrative, a description of general good health is offered to explain why the writer felt they should have been taken more seriously at triage:

'At one point I mentioned that it was 20 years since I last was off work sick. I'd assumed this would indicate I'm not a person to ask for help often or if I don't really need help. However, they interrupted to ask why that was relevant. I found that quite an astonishing question. I had already explained that I'm a self employed person and therefore not someone to be off work or asking for help or draw on resources if I don't definitely need help.' (Story from 2021, criticality rating 3)

Here, both good health and employment status are offered as evidence for the patient as someone to be treated respectfully, with an implied comparison with those who might often 'draw on resources'. The story goes on to describe staff resisting this evidence of virtue, and the patient being given pain medication and 'sent home': "I think they then said it was irrelevant when I'd last been off work sick and that the NHS is there to provide help when it's needed – which I heartily agreed with of course" (story from 2021, criticality rating 3). This story is largely one of frustration and unhappiness, and the decision to include this exchange, especially the appeal to common-sense ('of course'), are notable. The writer seems both committed to their starting point (that their broader lifestyle justifies being taken seriously) and particularly concerned to adhere to societal norms (that care is there when needed) as both patient and as narrator of patient experience.

A final, and often alternative route to presenting ones' narrative as that of a 'worthy' or 'proper' patient (Higashi et al, 2013) instead emphasises the heightened vulnerability of the patient. This was particularly prevalent where the writer was not the patient but their carer, and this was accentuated in the stories from 2021, where restrictions on access to hospital meant that carers could not always accompany vulnerable people as they might have usually. These narratives are sometimes written with a very purposeful effort to describe vulnerability in order to emphasise the importance of the narrative, for example: "Remember, she is alone, young and frightened" (story from 2019, criticality rating 0). This group of narratives often included the patient's specific age (as opposed to simply the descriptor 'elderly'): "My father is a 74-year-old man. He has had his health problems over the past few years including an abdominal aneurysm and a blood clot in his leg. He smoked for over 50 years and stopped abruptly 3 years ago and hasn't smoked since" (story from 2019, criticality rating 2).

As with earlier examples, narratives sometimes interwove vulnerability with virtue, including where patients had themselves worked in the NHS: "Elderly mother with multiple medical problems called local practice requesting help for chest infection and did not get past reception staff – was not even put on call back list. My mother had COPD and had worked as an NHS nurse for 40 years!" (story from 2021, criticality rating 3). Occasionally the descriptions are of the patient's own vulnerability: "My mother suffers from schizophrenia for the duration of my life and my father suffers from depression. I have told the doctors this. I need help. I'm not attention seeking. I have struggled for a very long time" (story from 2021, criticality rating 3). In this affecting example, intergenerational suffering is interwoven with descriptions of longstanding failures from the NHS to help.

It is worth emphasising that the Care Opinion platform doesn't prompt writers to provide these kinds of context. The prompts in the online form's free text box are simply 'What happened? How did you feel?' In my view, that so many stories provide context about how the patient accessed emergency care, about 'worthy patient' aspects of their conduct, and about the extreme need and vulnerability of patients, responds not just to medical power or dominance, but to the NHS context. As in Mazanderani et al's (2021) interviews on patient feedback: 'Understandings of how online feedback might improve healthcare were premised on pre-existing embodied, emotive and, at times ambivalent, relationships with the NHS.' Explicit and implicit logics of 'appropriate' or 'legitimate' service use held by both health professionals and patients are commonly identified in medical sociology studies (Hughes and Griffiths, 1997; Hillman, 2014; Llanwarne et al, 2017). It is significant, though, that in the narratives I analysed they are volunteered by patients and their carers. They suggest that, beyond a desire to be a 'good' patient in the face of medical power, patients seem to have an internalised awareness of attending A&E as drawing on a limited *public* resource. People explicitly referenced taking time, staff attention and beds 'away from' others in need. The 'good patient' is thus reconstructed as a good 'citizen-patient', and these details are repeatedly felt to be a necessary component of narratives of care.

When things go wrong: cushioning the blow

While gratitude was an overwhelming focus of the stories analysed, as several of these examples demonstrate, a range of narrative tactics were used in order to frame, cushion or justify negative descriptions within the stories. One key way people seemed to manage dissonance between their own experiences and a belief in the 'good' of the NHS is through blaming bad experiences on specific individuals rather than the NHS. This could at times conflict with the pervasive framing of NHS as 'heroes' or 'angels'.

> 'There was one doctor however who made the experience an unpleasant and upsetting one. Their bedside manner was poor and the way they talked to me and another patient across from me (whom I couldn't help but hear the way they spoke to him) was rude and to be honest shocking. They came to give me the results of the tests I'd undergone, during which time they came across as uncompassionate, uncaring and dismissive, suggesting my symptoms were down to anxiety.' (Story from 2021, criticality rating 3)

In stories such as this, where one health professional's behaviour is suggested to have sullied a whole experience, writers are often keen to balance their criticism with explicit descriptions of how *good* or kind other health professionals were. This acts both to present the writer as reasonable (a reliable narrator), and to suggest that something has gone wrong with the individual (in that other staff members managed to behave properly).

'Before I detail my concerns I must also state that throughout the past year I have experienced an incredible standard of care from the vast majority of the healthcare professionals I have come into contact with on my numerous journeys to and from hospital. Almost all of these people have treated me with huge amounts of empathy, kindness and delivered exemplary care with my comfort and dignity maintained as much as possible.' (Story from 2021, criticality rating 3)

It is possible that this specific tactic is related to the one-off nature of (many) emergency care interactions, in that patients in ongoing longer-term care pathways might feel more able to extend their assessment across a whole ward, department or even organisation. However within the emergency care narratives analysed, focusing criticism very specifically on individual staff members acts to insulate the broader NHS from criticism.

An alternative route to a similar outcome was to describe failures in care but to excuse them with reference to the notion of 'pressure' experienced by the NHS. At times the 'individual failure' is linked to this pressure:

'I include my long rambling story to illustrate the amazing machine the NHS is. So many pathways involved from start to finish during an incredibly pressurised time for the NHS. Only one example during my time of someone who was perhaps feeling the pressure and was a little uncaring. This is understandable. In 6 weeks I have gone from having pain to treatment and diagnosis. What a wonderful system.' (Story from 2021, criticality rating 2)

Noticeably, the prevalence of references to 'pressure' or 'pressures' is fairly consistent between 2019 and 2021, with the shock of the COVID-19 pandemic simply substituting for what, two years earlier, would have been references to government failure, underfunding or understaffing. Some 2021 stories did, though, ramp up the description of pressure from the COVID-19 pandemic as new and unique: "The pressure the NHS is under just now it's totally unprecedented and never in our lifetime has it ever been pushed to almost breaking point or never been so important to all of us. But break it didn't and I for one think this is incredible" (story from 2021, criticality rating 0). The pandemic context was extreme and many aspects of NHS delivery will have been unprecedented. Stories reflect that by using heightened language of pressure. But, comparing across multiple years, the *presence* of an external problem for which the NHS is blameless is a consistent feature.

In other stories, the 'pressure' is used to explain equanimity in response to quite startling breakdowns in care:

'He explained the theatres were backed up and it would be days before I'm seen ... I decided I could either take up bed space and cost to NHS to pity myself in hospital or put myself at home where I was more comfortable. Unfortunately this means a long waiting time before I get the treatment I need, this could all be behind me. Ninety per cent of the staff I came across gave you their full attention. Nothing was too much bother. It's so appreciated to have someone tell you that you aren't being dramatic and that you're suffering and they want to help. A few nurses were a little short tempered, but I suppose understandable with the pressure they're under.' (Story from 2021, criticality rating 1)

The longer story from which this is excerpt is taken, describes the painful exacerbation of a pre-existing problem requiring surgery. Despite the surgeons being willing to operate – 'this could all be behind me' – 'pressure' of capacity means that the patient decides to return home and await the surgical appointment for which they are already waiting. The alternative of taking up 'bed space and cost to NHS to pity myself in hospital' is rejected, and both this breakdown in sensible patient pathways and encounters with 'short-tempered' nurses is, somewhat reluctantly, attributed to 'the pressure they're under'. This story intrigues because the substantive content is of a frustrating, inefficient experience of the NHS, and yet the resolution is glowingly effusive about the staff encountered:

'These outstanding individuals will never know my gratitude. They stepped up patient after patient. They work tirelessly. I cannot thank them enough for being there during a very vulnerable time for me. Despite the sheer amount of patients, the fact they're under-funded as an institution and their physical exhaustion I was treated with the upmost care. Any problems were beyond their control and a result of the above issues.' (Story from 2021, criticality rating 1)

In this example, as in many others, external 'pressure' (underfunding in 2019, and then the COVID-19 pandemic in 2021) functions to create space for stories of failure to be told without criticising the NHS or (most of) its staff. At times, writers explicitly disavow the notion of complaining ("My only negative comment is that all but one of my face-to-face physio appointments have been cancelled but I totally understand why and make no complaint" [story from 2021, criticality rating 2]).

This broader search for a comfortable register in which to share negative stories is also reflected in stories where writers apologise for complaining. Several stories, especially where the writer is a current or past NHS employee, describe the *writers'* sadness at having to share negative experiences:

'I am very upset and sad to be writing this as I worked in NHS for 21 yrs and was always proud to work for NHS and the values and culture we all encouraged and upheld until this evening.' (Story from 2021, criticality rating 2)

'I am a nurse myself and I have always been proud of my profession however this evening I am sitting at home very upset and sad to have received the care I did.' (Story from 2021, criticality rating 2)

Each of these quotes emphasises the ambivalence of sharing negative feedback for the NHS, when one's identity as staff member is bound up with it. Other stories explicitly – if light-heartedly – apologise for complaining: "But every one of them – except one auxiliary! Sorry! – was a credit to the NHS. I am so grateful and full of admiration for all the work these people do every day" (story from 2019, criticality rating 0).

In another story, a patient seeking help for a suspected heart attack reflects on why their wife's requests for help weren't acknowledged:

'My wife had been out of cubicle a couple of times to try and get a doctor because I felt the heart attack coming on, I don't know if this was normal but I would not want to go back to that accident and emergency again if I had another heart attack, sorry to say you were too busy to notice my wife shouts or it wasn't your job I don't know.' (Story from 2019, criticality rating 2)

'Sorry to say' here is a sarcastic emphasis to this dangerous and upsetting experience, and even here, it is cushioned with the possible excuse that 'it wasn't your job'.

Conclusion

When analysing patient stories which invoke the NHS, I was struck by the recurrent phrasing 'I cannot fault' my care. As discussed, many of these stories are entirely positive, and 'I cannot fault it' is a colloquialism denoting everything being good, even perfect. However it also seems to speak to a broader discomfort of outright criticising care received in the NHS. It is important not to overstate this. Given the afore-mentioned particularities of Care Opinion, potentially actionable complaints are not likely to be featured in this corpus of data. Formal complaints, legal action and public inquiries into failures of care are all features of the UK system (Healthwatch, 2019; Department of Health, 2002; Ocloo, 2010). Despite many descriptions of problems within their care experiences, the authors of these stories had taken an active decision to take the time to write and share them. Rather than a taboo against naming failure, a more positive interpretation instead is that cushioned criticism stems from an active, even politicised, desire to protect the NHS from criticism while still offering feedback.

The analysis of patient narratives described suggests a struggle between the desire on the one hand to protect and support the NHS, and on the other to share difficult, at times traumatic experiences of care in order to hopefully improve care and bring about positive change. This tension is also evident in interview accounts of why people post online feedback (Mazanderani et al, 2021). In the stories analysed, people give credit to the NHS for good care given by people working within it, and attribute blame for failures in care, even devastating ones, to anywhere but the NHS. But, as Mazanderani et al (2021) report (from an interviewee), offering patient feedback is often prompted by a frustrated desire to be heard in order to effect change: "I felt that the NHS was not listening, that there was no way for me to talk to the NHS. I can't get the NHS in for a cup of coffee and say, 'Now look here NHS'" (quoted in Mazanderani et al, 2021, p 6).

This somewhat awkward personification of the NHS speaks to a desire for humanised healthcare, in which problems can be discussed openly, but the suggestion of sitting down over a hot drink also suggests a parallel concern to care *for* the NHS through feedback. As so often in this book, the NHS is imagined informally and fondly: this is neither church nor garage. The focus on things that need improvement evokes the way one might discuss an errant family member who needs to change their ways.

Other kinds of stories of service use might have offered a different picture of how affection for the NHS is intertwined with the embodied experience of seeking care. A focus on different clinical areas, including those where the NHS has particularly failed, might have yielded a more critical take on service use (Ocloo, 2010). As well as the particular emphases yielded by a focus on emergency care, the platform of Care Opinion will have shaped the narratives outlined. Formal complaints are one obvious alternative where the ideas I posit about credit and blame might be writ large, or entirely disproved (Reader, Gillespie and Roberts, 2014; Martin, Chew and Dixon-Woods, 2021). Another might be 'opting out', where people turn to private healthcare provision, frustrated or, especially given soaring waiting lists since the COVID-19 pandemic, unable to continue to wait for an appointment (Centre for Health and the Public Interest, 2022). In 2022, polling by Ipsos MORI reported that 13 per cent of respondents already paid for private healthcare, and a further 23 per cent stated they would be likely to pay for it if needed (The Health Foundation and Ipsos, 2022b). Private routes to diagnosis are particularly likely to be employed in underserved clinical areas such as Attention Deficit Hyperactivity Disorder, where NHS services are uneven and can constitute a 'postcode lottery' (Young et al, 2021).

Broader debates rage over the veracity and reliability of patient narratives of healthcare (Edwards, Staniszewska and Crichton, 2004; Shapiro, 2011). Managerial logics which require the standardisation of patient experiences, including complaints, in order to render them amenable to aggregation and 'action' (Edwards, Staniszewska and Crichton, 2004; Reader et al, 2014), are ill-suited to the complexity and breadth of many patient stories. Such efforts misunderstand some of the work that storytelling does in making sense of the heightened experience of vulnerability that is innate in many healthcare interactions. Shapiro (2011) argues, simply, that 'patients tell the stories they need to tell'. For the purposes of this book, I need no confirmation that these stories have a particular relationship to 'what really happened'. This makes the task both simpler, and more expansive. Shapiro argues that 'a patient's story is rarely "just a story"': 'People do not simply pull their narratives out of the blue, but in fact are deeply constrained by the power of the dominant narrative conventions and meta-narratives that are most readily available to them as a result of their particular place in time, history, culture and society' (Shapiro, 2011, p 69). Like all patient narratives, Care Opinion stories are 'inseparable from their cultural context' (Lucius-Hoene, Holmberg and Meyer, 2018). In this chapter I have explored the dominant meta-narratives evident in how we talk about our experiences of the NHS: gratitude, constructive criticism, and a concern with the legitimacy and reasonableness of our own claims on the system. My suggestion is that these tendencies in patient feedback are more than an unarticulated instinctive taboo for story writers as they respond to their socio-cultural context (Brookes et al, 2022). Rather, these are actively sought out opportunities to offer feedback as a gift to the NHS, and as such, are not merely cultural but also political acts.

7

What we can do with love: the future of the NHS in public

This is a difficult moment to be writing about the NHS, and especially to be pondering 'love' while the headlines are full of stories of harm and loss. Perhaps there is never a right moment: Klein has argued that the history of the NHS is 'punctuated by crises' (Klein, 2013). Chronicling decades of panic about the NHS's imminent demise, Powell (2015) wrote 'accounts of the death of the NHS have been exaggerated'. Yet, the consequences of a long spell of austerity coupled with the first global pandemic of the service's history makes this period of crisis particularly unsettling. This morning my radio alarm woke me with a news story about a woman named Koulla Mechanikos, who waited 14 hours for an ambulance to arrive when she broke her hip, and then 26 further hours in the ambulance to be brought into A&E (BBC News Online, 2022). Paton (2022) describes the current moment as a 'toxic cocktail': 'Austerity, the pandemic, Brexit, and barely sorted social care.' All this is to say, that for many of those working within or trying to use healthcare services in the UK, assertions of public love are likely to feel either irrelevant or, as others have argued (Arnold-Forster and Gainty, 2021), actively unhelpful.

And yet even as the material realities of healthcare feel pressing, I return to the importance of understanding 'the specific manner in which, at a given moment and in a specified society, the individual interaction between the doctor and the sick person is articulated upon the collective intervention with respect to illness in general' (Foucault, 2014). The NHS model makes that individual interaction between patient and healthcare system particularly public in nature. Investigating the affective formation of the NHS can be a route into the indistinct but pervasive elements of public discourse about healthcare in the UK, including some of the meta-narratives – gratitude, pride, exceptionalism – that perplex observers who are better versed in questions of comparative healthcare performance. Public discourse in the UK rarely emphasises the sheer value for money (or 'parsimony' (Berwick, 2008)) which is, in comparative terms, probably the most exceptional thing about the NHS (Papanicolas et al, 2019). Public attitudes to the NHS can be influential because of, and not despite, their fuzziness: 'a form of collectively held unconscious ideal which enacts meaning in codified rather than explicit ways, highlighting some ideas and obfuscating others' (Hunter, 2016, p 163).

The starting point of exploring public love for the NHS runs the risk of yielding a saccharine picture. Other key analyses of public discourse around the NHS focus on unpicking the consequences of a series of government policies and political campaigns: the Health and Social Care Act 2012; the co-optation of claims about the NHS in the campaign to leave the EU; the introduction of an inequitable NHS 'migrant surcharge' for non-citizens already subject to general taxation; and the more aggressive policing of fees incurred by non-residents for healthcare (Hunter, 2016; Fitzgerald et al, 2020). Grounded in these empirical realities of the contemporary NHS, a residual commitment to the NHS as progressive and solidaristic can seem naïve. However, rooting this book's analysis in public practices, rather than in policy, complicates such a resolutely critical stance. Public efforts to care for and contest the future of the NHS are often grounded in lofty ideals about solidarity, which seem still to hold remarkable power (Béland and Lecours, 2005; Prainsack and Buyx, 2017). More to the point, this chapter wants to argue that their persistence offers a potential route to a better, and fairer healthcare system. The time, energy and creativity that members of the public devote to the practices described in this book are significant. Beyond 'weepy sentiment' (Fitzgerald et al, 2020), 'nationalistic folktales' (Cowan, 2021) or 'irrational emotional pull' (Gorsky, 2008), I want to argue for these practices as an asset for improving health, not blindly loving a flawed system. In this chapter I recap the four practices of care and contestation discussed earlier in the book and explicate the way in which public love for the NHS is affective and cultural, but also political and material. I then go on to unpick two apparently dysfunctional consequences of the NHS's current public role: the NHS as a 'national identity', and (in public spending terms) the NHS 'on a pedestal'. Finally, I propose why an analysis of the ways we love the NHS might be a useful one, and offer a tentatively hopeful account of what else we might do with that love.

Practices of care and contestation

In this book I have offered an account of public love for the NHS since 2010 that weaves together 'the complex and rich meanings which the NHS holds for British publics: as family myth, personal life-saver, community supporter, or source of national identity' (Crane, 2022). The empirical content of the chapters centred on social practices: regularised patterns of interaction with the NHS which, while 'reinforced by visible symbols and ritual representations' (Barnes, 1993, p 215), are not external and unchanging but built and rebuilt in the everyday through people's actions. We learn how and when to be a patient (or a volunteer, campaigner or fundraiser) from those around us and then as we perform these roles, we strengthen these norms and thus shape the behaviour of those around us. Their effects can therefore intensify over time: even becoming 'interaction rituals, which generate a collective emotional energy that serves to imbue symbols with deepened cultural meanings' (Rossner and Meher, 2014). This book's assertion is that these practices collectively enact love for the NHS. That is, people often understand their 'appropriate' service use, fundraising, volunteering and campaigning as motivated by the ideal of the NHS, even when the experience reveals the NHS's disappointing or 'failing' aspects.

In Chapter 2, I used the concept of epistemic infrastructure to review the public opinion data that is the bedrock of policy and media debates about public views on the NHS. I demonstrated that these debates are overwhelmingly oriented to the more limited frame of 'satisfaction' with the NHS, with relatively little traction to understand more solidaristic or affective visions of the healthcare system. I additionally noted the way that sample sizes here limit what can robustly be concluded about variation in views across population groups, especially ethnic minority populations. I explored the community of organisations through which these simplifications (of both population and of phenomenon of interest) regularly make the front pages of national newspapers. Finally, drawing on critical takes on the public opinion industry creating 'opinioned' people (Osborne and Rose, 1999), I argued that the existence and substantial coverage of these data do not merely report but shape Britain's sense of itself as an 'opinioned' (Osborne and Rose, 1999) country that 'loves' its healthcare system.

Chapter 3 turned to an example with lengthy roots that has experienced a remarkable resurgence since the beginning of the COVID-19 pandemic: charitable fundraising for the NHS. The possibilities of charitable donations in the NHS have always existed, with somewhat fuzzy restrictions about their uses supplementing, and not replacing statutory spend by providing enhanced patient and staff amenities, as well as some medical equipment. However, the prevalence and scale of these efforts were suddenly and dramatically expanded by NHS Charities Together's Urgent COVID-19 Appeal. Presenting an analysis of the text content of 945 fundraising pages created by members of the public, I showed the extent to which these were oriented to gratitude towards staff as 'NHS heroes', but also how they mobilised broader narratives of national pride and solidarity in 'our NHS'. Building on the reach and ease of creating appeals on the GoFundMe and JustGiving platforms (Kenworthy, 2021), this appeal generated a new mode of mass participation in loving the NHS during an exceptional moment of health emergency (Stewart et al, 2022).

Chapter 4 explored another facet of charitable activity in the NHS which has received a lot of policy attention, but commensurately *less* academic research; members of the public volunteering within NHS organisations.

I explore experiences of volunteering in hospitals, demonstrating how, especially in smaller community hospitals which are deeply embedded in their communities (Davidson et al, 2019), volunteering is often based on long-term relationships. Volunteers described it as relatively informal and changing over time, negotiated between the interests and skills of potential volunteers and the openness of management to their contributions. While motivations are complex to unpick, I argued that doing 'a good thing', and also the pleasures of social connection, dominate volunteers' descriptions of why they give their time to the NHS. I also compared these examples with a flurry of national 'branded' NHS volunteering schemes that launched before and during the early pandemic outpouring of affection for the NHS, and reflected on the ways in which these quasi-militaristic calls for service might reflect a new era of NHS volunteering.

Chapter 5 considered examples of public campaigning in and about the NHS, including local campaigns to save or protect hospitals threatened with closure, and two left-wing national campaigns: Keep our NHS Public and Save our NHS. Comparing these local and national mobilisations – which are also linked to each other – sheds light on different frames of what needs protecting in the NHS. Specifically, local campaigns orient to what is special about their specific institutions of care, while national campaigns link examples of patient experience much more tightly to the founding principles of the NHS: especially to universal access to healthcare, free at the point of use. This analysis emphasises the preservationist character of these campaigns, particularly when compared to the more radical and change-oriented campaigning Crane has identified as the advent of national NHS campaigning in the 1980s (Crane, 2019, 2022). This suggests that contemporary campaigning, while still centring progressive aspects of Britain's healthcare system, focuses more explicitly on nostalgia for an NHS that is perceived to have been degraded (Cowan, 2021), than proposing specific reforms. This shift in emphasis risks making it more difficult to identify problems and things about healthcare in the UK that *should* change, especially longstanding issues that are not only a consequence of straitened funding (Arnold-Forster and Gainty, 2021; Cowan, 2021).

Chapter 6 shifts towards the terrain of medical sociology, by considering the ways in which affection for the NHS shape embodied experiences of healthcare in the UK. This builds on an analysis of patient feedback on experiences of emergency medicine in the UK that were submitted to the Care Opinion website in 2019 and in 2021, in which the authors made reference to 'the' NHS or 'our' NHS. These are, of course, a self-selected sample of experiences, but especially given the consumeristic origins of Care Opinion as an information tool for the quasi-market era of the English NHS, the overall positivity of stories is striking. Significant numbers of patients use Care Opinion simply to thank their care-givers, often adding gratitude to 'the NHS' alongside identifying specific health professionals who are perceived as having gone 'above and beyond'. I identify the way in which negative experiences recounted are softened, blamed on individuals or presented as constructive, and the effort to which authors go to present themselves as a legitimate narrator and patient. I argue that these features are not only a consequence of medical hierarchies – the desire to perform a legitimate 'sick role' – but are imbued with the particular characteristics of NHS care. This, I suggest, entails that one's own claims on the system, and the system's response, are understood as qualified entitlements, in relation to the ability of the system to meet all the claims made upon it. Thus the persistent and consistent references within these narratives to the NHS as 'under pressure': whether pressure of budget cuts or of the century's first pandemic, using the NHS is understood as making demands on a finite system.

Towards a multi-dimensional understanding of love for the NHS

This book resists the temptation to offer a singular and definitive answer to the question of how Britain loves the NHS. I offer instead an analysis of a series of practices, as lenses through which to understand this multi-dimensional relationship.

Practices of this kind aren't intrinsically good or bad. They need to be assessed in context and with a view to both their immediate consequences and their broader impact on the healthcare system. Recent analyses have emphasised the way that public valorisation of the NHS has shaped a context for regressive political campaigns, which play on the symbolic value of the NHS in UK society (Hunter, 2016; Fitzgerald et al, 2020). This book builds on these insights to explore the way in which public practices of love are also acts of agency: asserting that the practices of care and contestation that contribute to Britain's love for the NHS need to be understood as affective and cultural, but also as material and political. This argument resonates with recent calls from social policy theorists for better acknowledgement of public roles as 'doers' and 'judges', as well as 'receivers', within welfare states (Bonvin and Laruffa, 2022).

This book's empirical chapters underline the *affective* significance of the NHS in UK society: 'The ways in which emotion works through culture as the connective tissue of institutional life' (Hunter, 2016). This book centres a broadly-conceived vision of love, and its societal (re)enactment, rather than satisfaction (the meeting of consumeristic standards of quality). This better explains how deeply held attachments to the NHS seem to be, and the role that ideas of the NHS play in moments of crisis (Day et al, 2022) and celebration (Thomson, 2022). And yet engaging seriously with affect also forces us to move beyond simply noting that fact. While consumeristic satisfaction is grounded in satisfaction with one's own, or perhaps one's loved one's care, the practices described in this book often attributed love for the NHS to a, possibly naïve hope that everyone 'we share this country with' will be taken care of. This is the pride that is referenced repeatedly in patient narratives, in campaign texts and fundraising appeals. It is part, in Hunter's analysis of discourse around the NHS, of a 'more complicated multicultural national fantasy which … protects against a related set of (post)colonial anxieties … which deepen in the context of austerity politics and dwindling financial resources' (Hunter, 2016).

These practices described contribute to the currently intensified *cultural* role of the NHS in society. Many of the chapters depict campaigns seeking to enrol broader publics into the NHS: whether recruiting volunteers, opposing reforms, soliciting donations or requesting feedback on patient experience. These build a sense of 'the NHS' not as organisation but as a collective national project. In his analysis of the mundane practices through which 'the state' has effects, Painter depicts

> the intensification of the symbolic presence of the state across all kinds of social practices and relations. Again, this does not mean that real institutions are not involved; courts, police, schools, councils and so on all exist. But whether their activities constitute statisation depends on the nature of the practices in which they are engaged, not on the categorization of any particular institution as a part of the state or not. Thus, statisation can occur through practices undertaken by nominally non-state organizations, such as private businesses. (Painter, 2006, p 758)

Thus an intensified cultural role for the NHS – as experienced in the omnipresence of NHS branding since the COVID-19 pandemic – can be built on appeals and campaigns from non-NHS organisations. Not only NHS charities, but private companies donating to them, the *Daily Mail* newspaper and, of course, the profit-making companies who delivered 'NHS Test and Trace' as part of the country's COVID response under NHS branding (Mahase, 2021) contribute to the intensification. Members of the public who respond positively to these campaigns are further embedded into the affective formation of the contemporary NHS. These practices generate new opportunities for 'supporting the NHS' to become an available and appealing social, and perhaps even national, identity.

The analysis offered in this book also suggests that publics hold, and enact, their views on the NHS more strategically and *politically* than much literature allows. Enacting love for the NHS into practices and statements has created a context where it is at least surprising, and in some corners actively taboo, to criticise the NHS (Hunter, 2016; Arnold-Forster and Gainty, 2021). This can give NHS love a culturally hegemonic character. However this book showcases practices of both care and contestation, not merely uncritical celebration (Crane, 2022). Commitment to what the NHS is perceived to stand for, and not simply blind or mistaken loyalty, I would suggest, explains the somewhat hyperbolic 77 per cent of people in England polled in 2017 who agreed with the statement that 'the NHS is crucial to British society and we must do everything we can to maintain it' (Ipsos MORI for the King's Fund, 2017). The enthusiasm with which people enrol in practices of support for the NHS, and the reluctance to name unacceptable instances of care demonstrated in Chapter 6, are political, as well as blindly affective acts. Significantly, they come in a context of near continual crisis – actual and perceived (Duncan, 1998; Powell, 2015). Even in periods where it was more robustly funded and satisfaction was high, the NHS has never not been seen as a problem to be solved. As a national health system it is a visible and explicit site for contestation, in which competing visions of society are played out.

However the NHS is additionally a set of institutions in which bodies and minds are treated, cups of tea are handed out, and in which people are born and die. The approach taken in this book re-emphasises these *material* dimensions of the NHS as institution. Hunter's conceptualisation of the affective formation of the NHS acknowledges its material existence, but in its focus on political discourse, neglects the particular embodied encounters that ground the daily 'technical, bureaucratic and professional' (Hunter, 2016) realities of healthcare systems. This book accentuates *medical* material realities both in the descriptions of service use in Chapter 6, but also in people's descriptions of service use within the broader range of public acts of support for it. I reassert the significance of these material encounters, which are often downplayed in health system analyses. In his ode to NHS care, *Many Different Kinds of Love*, Rosen describes readers' surprise at the 'very basic and visceral' descriptions in the book: 'That's where you get to sometimes: just you, in your body, with your body' (Rosen, 2021, p 301). Medical encounters need not be romanticised for us to acknowledge their significance. The King's Fund estimates that in 2020 in England alone, on an average day 1 million people had a GP appointment and nearly 45,000 would attend an A&E department (The King's Fund, 2022). These can be converted into 'units of activity', tracked and plotted onto graphs for evaluative dissection. But they can also be understood as moments in people's lives which are unusually likely to matter 'existentially' (Freeman, 2008): 'For the typical physician, my illness is a routine incident in his rounds, while for me it's the crisis of my life' (Broyard, 1992, p 43).

These near universal experiences of the intensely significant and intimate nature of healthcare – identifying a problem, seeking help from healthcare professionals, receiving care – are in the UK NHS rendered particularly public (Sturdy, 2002). We can see this in the increasing prevalence of campaigns to ask people to make more healthy lifestyle choices, and to use services more 'appropriately'. But, as every chapter of this book demonstrates, it is also a connection made by members of the public when they 'defend' the NHS. The analysis of Chapter 6 suggests a possibly counter-intuitive role for increased media coverage of NHS failures, as patients gratefully attribute positive experiences of care to 'the NHS' and search for someone *else* to blame for experienced failures.

Better recognising the affective, cultural, material and political dimensions of how Britain loves the NHS also illuminates the multidimensional nature of people in society: as 'receivers' with vulnerabilities; as 'doers' with meaningful contributions to make; and as 'judges', with aspirations and a right to voice (Bonvin and Laruffa, 2022).

What love does

The practices explored in this book are thus prompted by, and also generate, particular forms of public affection in the NHS. In this section I consider two sets of political consequences of the current configuration of how Britain loves the NHS. One is the manner in which the NHS increasingly stands in as a proxy for a substantive national identity. The second is a perception that the NHS is, politically, on a pedestal when it comes to public sector funding, driving the rolling back of broader social protection and other forms of public investment.

As discussed earlier, during the height of the COVID-19 pandemic, effusive expressions of gratitude for the NHS were front and centre: signs stuck in windows, clapping on doorsteps, and raising money for NHS charities (and talking about doing so on social media). Sociologist Gary Younge's astute writing in newspaper columns during the COVID-19 pandemic repeatedly called attention to the apparent emptiness of these celebrations of the NHS and carers: these activities were, he stated, a 'meme in pursuit of a meaning' (Younge, 2020). Remarkably, Nye Bevan identified this risk 70 years earlier when he wrote that social institutions (such as the NHS): 'Are what they do, not necessarily what we say they do. It is the verb that matters, not the noun. If this is not understood, we become symbol worshippers' (Bevan, 2010).

Ironically, Bevan's quote-worthy rhetoric is often incorporated into symbolic celebrations of the NHS. One can buy tea towels with significant Bevan quotes: I was given one last Christmas. Witness: 'A free Health Service is a triumphant example of the superiority of collective action and public initiative applied to a segment of society where commercial principles are seen at their worst' (Bevan, 2010). Both Hansen (2022) and Meer (2022) note the strong resemblance between contemporary valorisation of the NHS, and the tenor of Bevan's early speeches on the topic. The narratives of British exceptionalism that Bevan (2010) featured are, we can now recognise, predicated on Britain's role as a violent coloniser and a ruthless extractor of wealth from other populations around the world (Sanghera, 2021; Bhambra, 2022a; Hansen, 2022). Bhambra demonstrates that this is not only a question of the national stories we tell about ourselves: the NHS was financed and staffed through the extractive work of empire (Bhambra, 2022a; Millar, 2022). The seduction of soaring rhetoric about the NHS remains. Sixty years later, behold American healthcare improvement guru Don Berwick in a conference speech: 'Cynics beware, I am romantic about the National Health Service; I love it. All I need to do to rediscover the romance is to look at health care in my own country. The NHS is one of the astounding human endeavours of modern times' (Berwick, 2008). The healthcare system's residual grounding in solidaristic goals (Prainsack and Buyx, 2017) gives it an apparent simplicity as a rallying cry. As a symbolic national 'achievement', the NHS thus offers a meeting point for a far broader coalition of people than more obviously complicated national institutions like the monarchy or the military.

Valorisation of the NHS is also rooted in what Younge depicts as the evasiveness of notions of British identity: 'British identity has no lodestar; it is grounded in no principle; put bluntly it has no point beyond its own self-assertion' (Younge, 2022). There are, as Younge acknowledges, differences in national sentiment across the UK, with the imagined communities of Scotland, Wales and Northern Ireland often defined *against* a notion of Britishness. For the rest of the UK population, its overwhelming majority, the substance of English national identity is more complex. It is intriguing that, in this context, the NHS branding of volunteering programmes (as discussed in Chapter 4) and the concerned policing of the NHS brand identity (as described in Chapter 1) are particularly features of the context in England, and less apparent in the smaller devolved healthcare systems. Henderson and Jones (2021, p 4) argue that English national identity 'combines a sense that England has been "forgotten" and unfairly submerged, with the belief that Britain, self-evidently, is or should be, should be, "the greatest nation on earth"'. The NHS as national achievement can stand in here, for 'greatness', but also just for *something* to unite around. In her study of the social roles of happiness, Ahmed proposes: 'We might have a social bond if the same objects make us happy. I am suggesting here that happiness itself can become the shared object' (Ahmed, 2010, p 56). This might explain the way in which loving the NHS (or thanking or celebrating it) can become connective, while increasingly detached from the material realities of healthcare delivery.

It is in this context that the 'weepy sentiment' (Fitzgerald et al, 2020) of love for the NHS looks particularly suspicious: a sop for the masses to distract from their plight. The NHS can be imagined as one of the 'system of ditches to protect capitalism and hegemonic groups' (Filc, 2014, p 170). However a Gramscian notion of cultural hegemony around the NHS is not entirely convincing. First, the material realities of healthcare delivery continue to intrude into people's lives, not as symbols but as bloody, or scary, or debilitating moments in our lives. Second, the power bases of the

NHS, the hegemonic groups, are multiple and disunited. While policy actors certainly imagine and seek particular roles for the population at particular times, the practices described in this book are also active ways for members of the public to contest and enact possible NHS futures (Fortier, 2016). The notion of the NHS from church to garage (Klein, 2013) was always, of course, something of a caricature, and it was focused on the population as policy audience, not as actors. Centring public love for the NHS, through practices of both care and of contestation, means that neither church nor garage feels apt. The remarkable contemporary ascendance of discourses about 'our NHS' denotes something less sacred than a church; yet still more collectivist and affectively significant than a garage. The research in this book suggests that the NHS is often seen as a fragile, crisis-prone yet shared achievement, which we all have a part to play in protecting. All four practices explored in this book have in common an orientation as active stakeholders in, and not mere customers nor congregation of, the NHS.

A second macro-level political consequence of perceived public love for the NHS relates to public spending. During her 2022 Conservative party leadership campaign, Liz Truss argued that the NHS must face the same budget cuts she planned to make across the gamut of state spending. On 20 August, *The Guardian*'s frontpage headline was 'NHS "cannot be put on a pedestal" – Truss' (Mason, 2022). This claim, based on a thinktank pamphlet Truss co-authored in 2009 before entering Parliament, was frontline news because, while it became commonplace under the Conservative government to claim to 'protect' NHS spending from broader cuts, this explicit use of the pedestal metaphor went further. It invokes the idea that Britain's glorification of its health service, rather than an evidence-based decision, has prompted its relative protection from broader austerity government. In a *Spectator* article to promote the pamphlet, Truss is quoted as stating:

> We have identified £30 bn cuts across the 'big five'; defence, health, work & pensions, communities and education. … No department can be a no go area. This means the NHS, accounting for a sixth of government expenditure, cannot be put on a pedestal. Doctors' pay which has risen inexorably needs to be restrained. Superfluous bodies such as Strategic Health Authorities, and health campaigns exhorting the public to stop 'vegging out', should be abandoned. (Quoted in Mason, 2022)

While Truss's suggestion of where healthcare funding has gone is dubious, the NHS has indeed been spared some of the most swingeing funding cuts that have been made to the welfare state since the 2010s. Having received significant funding increases during the New Labour era, the NHS has experienced what is referred to as 'funding restraint' since 2010 (Edwards,

2022a). While not enough, say many commentators, to support an ageing and growing population, this is less disastrous than in related areas such as social care services (mostly funded by local government) or working age benefits. It is true that broader public spending has been more savagely cut than NHS budgets, especially spending on social protection (Farnsworth, 2021) and local government budgets (Gray and Barford, 2018).

The NHS is not *only* cushioned from the worst of funding cuts by perceived public support for it, but this support is often powerfully intertwined with other protective factors. The counterfactuals of healthcare (what if there was no NHS) feel more immediate and visible than policy areas whose benefits are more diffuse and long term. Internationally, Jensen emphasises the 'special importance ascribed to health care in modern-day societies, where other physical risks have been mainly eliminated; in a very real sense, the risk of poor health is universal and therefore provides a strong political motive for public health care provision' (Jensen, 2008, p 160). Public spending on healthcare can, as discussed earlier, be the 'acceptable face' of public spending because much (although not all) need for healthcare is less stigmatised than need for, for example, social security benefits (Wendt et al, 2010; Carpenter, 2012). While the British Social Attitudes Survey consistently puts levels of public support for services (that is, healthcare and education), above public support for benefits, support for spending on healthcare in particular increased during the pandemic (de Vries et al, 2020). As discussed earlier in this book, the deceptive appearance of unity and simplicity of 'the NHS' as a brand can be a particularly powerful symbol.

Another cushioning effect is that healthcare and state governance are often particularly intertwined: hence Moran's (1999) concept of the 'healthcare state'. Health professionals, particularly doctors, have both an unusual proximity to the state (which often governs their professional registration), and through those processes of professional registration, a 'natural basis of organisation' (Carpenter, 2012, p 298). Even if medical autonomy has been squeezed (Harrison and Ahmad, 2000), health professional associations remain powerful actors in UK health politics, and health professionals have both official governmental roles (such as Chief Medical Officers) and significant cultural capital (Greer, 2004). Professional power is thus often buoyed by its status among the broader public, and this status was further boosted by the focus on 'NHS heroes' during the COVID-19 pandemic (Cox, 2020).

None of this is to suggest that the NHS is in an enviable position within the welfare state. The current crisis shows how unhelpful this cushioning can be. The relative protection of the NHS is short-sighted, as well as politically cynical, because of a series of upstream causes of ill-health. Our understanding of healthcare has moved far from the curative model on which the NHS was built (Darlington-Pollock, 2022; Greener, 2022). As other kinds of social support fail, people turn up at the NHS's door with more intractable problems. The health consequences of cutbacks on education budgets turn up at the door of Child and Adolescent Mental Health Services. The health consequences of a punitive, suspicious benefits system turn up in GP waiting rooms. And, as any semblance of a social care system crumbles, hospitals fill with people who cannot go home without care services, and ambulances queue at the front door, unable to discharge patients needing care. Economists often argue that the NHS needs increases in funding year-on-year just to stand still (Charlesworth and Bloor, 2018). They are right, but if the other preventative planks of wellbeing in society are removed, there is no proportionate increase in NHS funding that can bridge the gap. In their efforts to find solutions healthcare professionals will often, as they are trained to do, medicalise the issues. They might even 'prescribe' social solutions to the issues people present with, drawing on local ecosystems of voluntary organisations (Tierney et al, 2020). But the NHS cannot solve these problems while other parts of the welfare state are broken, and, of course, it is manifestly unable to prevent them from occurring in the first place.

What (else) we can do with love

While for Arnold-Forster and Gainty (2021) public love for the NHS is to be abandoned as an obstacle to reform, on balance I disagree. This might well be because my research locates me mostly in the public realm, rather than in clinical spaces where inequalities in care are more starkly evident (Cowan, 2020). However it is mostly because, with a background in the discipline of social policy, I have residual faith in the potential of a solidaristic upsurge of affect around the NHS (Titmuss, 2004; Prainsack and Buyx, 2017). These sorts of not-strictly rational, deeply felt sentiments are what sustain public services (Bambra et al, 2021; Cooper and Burchardt, 2022). They are only intrinsically problematic if we assume that healthcare is a consumer industry like any other, rather than a complex system of interrelated vulnerabilities and capabilities which the broader public is part of, in myriad and complex ways (Cribb, 2018). That the NHS fails sometimes, and that the population famously 'loves' it, doesn't mean that there is a causal link in either direction between the two. Nigel Edwards, Chief Executive of the Nuffield Trust, recently wrote an essay 'myth-busting' the idea that public affection prevents necessary reforms of the NHS (Edwards, 2022b). Indeed, he argued that the NHS had been too frequently reformed, but that the problem has been that these are poorly-planned, national and top-down reorganisations in an effort to win party political points.

Much recent concern about Britain's love for the NHS relates to the discomforts of how it has been co-opted into a narrow nationalism in the run up to and aftermath of Brexit. Stanley (2022) describes how the project of 'austerity' since 2008 has included a renationalising of the NHS, as access to care for non-UK citizens was made more difficult and costly due to overseas patient charging and the Migrant Health Surcharge. However, and inspired by Cowan's call to find 'better ways to put this care, love, and energy to use' (Cowan, 2020, p 214), I want to consider how we might make collective affection for the NHS more generative. The practices of care and contestation explored in this book cohere comfortably with Cribb's call for a shift from 'an assumed model of "top-down" service delivery towards a more diffuse and democratic model' (Cribb, 2018, p 153). Imagining a future for the NHS which neither ignores nor becomes complacent to its current failings, but seeks to learn from them, seems not only worthwhile but vital. After all, every society needs a way to meet the healthcare needs of its population. My suggestion is that we take seriously that public affection for the NHS is predicated on its offer of universality: 88 per cent of those in 2021 polling claim to agree with this 'founding principle' (The Health Foundation and Ipsos, 2022a). I want to posit the possibility that we can have a mature, open conversation about what it would take to make that meaningful. One set of possibilities here relates to reimagining public roles in the NHS, and another linked one is to challenge Britain's professed emotional commitment to universal care for all to build a more constructive public conversation about the broader welfare state.

Despite decades of effort towards 'public and patient involvement', the story of the NHS remains overwhelmingly a power battle between government and clinical bodies (Klein, 2013; Newbigging, 2016). The last decade of the expansion of the rhetoric of 'our NHS' has not been significantly accompanied by changes to enable collective, rather than individualistic, empowerment in healthcare in any of the constituent parts of the NHS (Newbigging, 2016). However, there is cause for hope. The empirical chapters of this book support existing evidence that there is public appetite to play more active roles in the NHS than passive consumer (Newman and Clarke, 2009). Calls for more dialogic approaches to improvement and decision-making (Cribb, 2018) have potential to generate many more opportunities for debate and engagement. At organisational level, new possibilities are already being carved out. Formal roles of patient leadership with people with significant experience of using health services are increasingly seen as mainstream, if not yet widely operationalised (Gilbert, 2019). Integration of health and social care services has prompted more connections with local government, so that elected representatives should have greater oversight of services (Reed et al, 2021). The thinktank *New Local*'s vision of a Community-powered NHS also offers new ideas, based on more meaningful localism and participation in the NHS, each of which deserve more attention (Lent, Pollard and Studdert, 2022).

On the other hand, after a decade in which the NHS 'brand' has become increasingly prominent, it might also be time for more national-level dialogue about the future of the NHS within the UK's constituent parts. In 2012, NHS England created a remarkably ambitious experiment in systemic deliberation, which, while it currently (NHS England, 2022b) appears to have floundered back into the realms of 'committee work' (Stewart, 2016), did at least for a while acknowledge the possibility of recognising collective citizen voice as a priority (Dean, Boswell and Smith, 2019). Recent efforts to develop meaningful proposals for reform of social security (Commission on Social Security, 2022) and of social care (Social Care Future, 2022) with lived experience at its centre, might inspire a resurgence of what often feels a staid, entrenched debate about the future of the NHS. Building on public expressions of love and gratitude for the NHS to identify shared priorities seems to have great potential for a refreshed public debate about the NHS, as the rather brief report from the King's Fund's small commissioned discussion groups suggested (Ewbank et al, 2018). That challenges the assumption that public demand for more, better and more expensive medicine is limitless, as does the evidence in this book of a 'stakeholder' orientation to services from at least some of the population. Recent initiatives in Scotland towards Realistic Medicine and Wales towards Prudent Medicine both showed a path towards a more parsimonious future which nonetheless prioritised equity of access (Bradley et al, 2014; NHS Scotland, 2015). These agendas were, though, clinically led with minimal attention to broader engagement: as so often, the NHS waits to 'sell' its vision to the public after decisions are made (Greer et al, 2021). But each could have been, and perhaps still could be, a meaningful opportunity to start from population perspectives and build a sustainable NHS, especially while paying better attention to the experiences of under-represented groups including ethnic minorities and immigrants. In this, the devolved nations with their vastly smaller populations surely have an easier task on their hands. These solutions are all, it should be noted, collective ones in which the population are partners. This pragmatically recognises the way in which we have come to understand that health and wellbeing are located not in hospitals but in people's daily lives. It is also a normative one, which acknowledges that democratic solutions to public problems are rooted in our interdependence (Cribb, 2018).

Beyond just realising the vision of 'our NHS', we can consider building on this public affection as a starting point for a much broader defence of the welfare state. Cooper and Burchardt's recent analysis of the British Social Attitudes Survey suggests that claims about the polarisation of attitudes to welfare, and the internalisation of discourses of austerity (Farnsworth, 2021), might have been overstated. They suggest that, in the aftermath of the pandemic, there is a moment of 'significant attitudinal capital' in which more progressive policies might be enacted (Cooper and Burchardt, 2022). There may be lessons in the rhetorical power the NHS seems to have on popular imaginations (Crane and Hand, 2022), and potential to expand it to broader ways that the welfare state cares for the population. Our understanding of healthcare's role in the welfare state has transformed dramatically since the creation of the NHS. In his reassessment of Beveridge's Five Giants, Greener (2022) proposes that 'preventable mortality', and not 'disease' should be the welfare state's target (see also Darlington-Pollock, 2022). Medical models of social problems tend to pursue expensive solutions through innovation and technology, because healthcare systems have relatively little realistic prospect of preventing problems at source. Indeed preventative care often descends into well-meaning but, in the long term, ineffective efforts at health promotion (Katikireddi et al, 2013). Reducing preventable mortality is overwhelmingly about broader structural changes to society (Pickett and Wilkinson, 2015; Bambra et al, 2021). Can we imagine a world where 'our JobCentre', 'our schools' and 'our social housing' are revered in a similar way to 'our NHS' as safety nets with societal benefits?

Conclusion

This book has reviewed the way that public support for the NHS is conceptualised and measured in UK debates, and proposed an alternative way forward that better illuminates the multiple ways that people in the UK encounter and value our sprawling healthcare system. I have argued that the epistemic infrastructures of quantitative data which structure our understanding of public love for the NHS struggle to capture the complexity of relationships involved. The baldness with which media reports proclaim the data reported in Chapter 2, and the relative lack of interest in how views about the NHS might be patterned in the population, are both obstacles to a better understanding of the NHS 'in public'. I offer this book as the beginning of a more curious and wide-ranging research agenda in this area, rather than as a done-and-dusted answer. The practices covered here are not a complete list of practices which might illuminate the relationship between population and healthcare system, but examples to illustrate the possibilities of this approach.

One of the most obvious candidates for further research is an exploration of how NHS staff, across the spectrum of roles, practise care and contestation for the NHS in their work. For example, (how) do those recently vaunted as 'NHS heroes' understand their working conditions and the 'above and beyond' work they do (see Chapter 6) as service to the NHS? In a context of industrial action (Issa and Butt, 2022) and staff activism (Pushkar and Tomkow, 2021), there is much more to understand about how being employed by the UK's biggest employer constitutes a particular positionality. Writing in the *British Medical Journal*, General Practitioner Margaret McCartney wrote of 'doctors and the serial devastation the UK's National Health Service (NHS) wrecks upon them' (McCartney, 2022). Six years earlier, her book on 'keeping the promise of the NHS' began 'I am furious, sad, and scared for the NHS' (McCartney, 2016). Working for the NHS is part of UK health professional identity, yet it is routine now to hear tales of NHS doctors uprooting their lives to make international moves for better remuneration and conditions in countries including Canada and Australia (Brennan et al, 2021). How, if at all, does commitment to the NHS feature in the sacrifices involved in staying, or in decisions to leave? And how are issues of overwork and underpay managed by those people and occupational groups who lack the possibility of international mobility?

Future research in this area also needs to be more purposively focused on particular population groups. I'm mindful, as I write and think about these issues, that the story of how 'Britain' feels about anything is one that only limited sections of its population (let alone the broader global population whose living conditions are structured by the former British empire), have been given space to narrate (Meer, 2022). Especially given the increasing co-optation of the NHS into particular visions of nationalism, it is especially pressing to understand whether and how diverse communities see the NHS not (only) as patients but as members of UK society. For example, many of the practices explored in this book are highly gendered, as well as being located within structures of social class, 'race' and migration status. The empirical studies reported in this book rely on convenience sampling in case study locations, and the overwhelming majority of my interviewees are white British, leaving multiple gaps in perspective. There is evidence that people who have migrated to the UK from other health systems are often less impressed by 'our wonderful NHS' than people raised in Britain proclaim ourselves to be (Madden et al, 2017; Bradby et al, 2020). Belatedly, important work is happening to understand and address experiences of racial discrimination in the NHS, and we know that experience of the NHS is sharply patterned by ethnicity (Black Equity Organisation and Clearview Research, 2022; NHS Race and Health Observatory, 2022). Experiences of healthcare systems are also different across other facets of identity: for example Lesbian, Gay, Bisexual and Transgender populations (Pearce, 2018; Young et al, 2019). Future research should prioritise better understanding how members of marginalised groups feel about 'the NHS', and how the increasing 'nationalisation' of the service (Cowan, 2021; Stanley, 2022) might be experienced from different subject positions.

There are thus multiple potential avenues to continue expanding and improving knowledge of public feelings about the NHS. This book is a beginning, rooted in the dissonance of watching symbolic statements of gratitude and love for the NHS proliferate, amid a broader feeling of crisis in 2021 and 2022. It really did feel, for a while, like 'thankyou NHS' was everywhere I went. In summer 2021, I took my kids to Legoland for a post-lockdown treat and took photos of them standing awkwardly in front of the 'thankyou NHS' exhibit in Miniland. At Christmas, my partner brought home a 'love NHS' advent calendar, with small pictures of the fundraiser Captain Tom Moore and rainbows all over it, with part of the purchase price being donated to NHS charities. I stepped off a train in Kings Cross railway station on my way to a London meeting, and the train pulling away from the next platform had 'thank you NHS' flashing on the digital screen instead of its destination. When I took my child for a hospital appointment, the ground outside the hospital had been emblazoned with a vast Thankyou NHS slogan, coloured in rainbow stripes. The data sources gathered in this book are testament to the intensification of Britain's love for the NHS that I experienced in this period. The NHS has a remarkable and, as Crane and Hand (2022) have shown, novel cultural role in the UK as we move into the aftermath of the COVID pandemic. This book is, I hope, the beginning of a better understanding of that role, in the hope that we might use it to fashion a better, and fairer, 'healthcare state' (Moran, 1999) for the future.

APPENDIX

Research methods

In this book, I employ a range of qualitative methods to explore public practices and discourses around love and the NHS. The toolbox I draw from is somewhat eclectic, combining 'found' data (which has been created by members of the public for other purposes), and 'generated' data (from research studies using a range of interviews and observation to build case studies). In this chapter I describe my methods in greater detail, for the purposes of transparency and openness, and to enable readers to form a judgement on the robustness of my findings (Mays and Pope, 2000). However, this chapter also offers reflections on my own positionality within the research overall. As a qualitative health researcher, I recognise that procedural requirements – what aspects of data collection and analysis to report and using what terms – are inadequate to the task of understanding my process and my claims in the round (Eakin and Mykhalovskiy, 2003). Such details, offered next, provide some of the context from which the data are drawn, but the vital and distinctively qualitative approaches of reflexivity and positionality are near impossible to communicate in formulaic lists. My approach as a researcher is rooted in feminist praxis which understands that the account I offer is inseparable from my own, personal perspective on this research. The stylistic detachment of many of the key texts on the NHS may be more effective in conveying gravitas, but in doing so it creates an unrealistic impression that the authors offer a 'view from nowhere' (Shaw et al, 2015).

Acknowledging my view from somewhere, and explaining how I have reflected on my own perspectives as I conduct research, are central to the approach of this book (Harding, 2004). This approach is reflected in the first-person writing style, in the incorporation of auto-ethnographic research in Chapter 6, and indeed in my linking up of data across multiple studies which I have designed and led. In carrying out research projects, analysing data and discussing with research participants and collaborators, I have brought my own knowledge of the UK NHS, not just acquired through research and study, but as a patient, carer and parent. This doesn't feel like a particularly authoritative standpoint within much discussion of healthcare (Rowland et al, 2017). As Arnold-Forster (2022) notes, the most influential or popular accounts of the NHS are produced by health professionals. I do this research and write this book not as an NHS insider or someone whose working life has been spent in hospitals. If friends who work in the NHS ask me about the book and I tell them the title, I always feel like a bit of a fraud. On the other hand I often wonder whether I am 'patient enough': that is, whether my (thus far, thankfully) fairly occasional service use qualifies me, whether I have enough of what David Gilbert, a patient leader and advocate describes as 'jewels of wisdom and insight that are dug from the caves of suffering' (Gilbert, 2019). Rather, I look at the NHS mostly from the outside, as a sort of long-term participant observer of its place in society.

That standpoint is also imbued with the privilege of whiteness in Britain. I am mindful that some of what seems harmless, if banal, about the NHS's increasing nationalisation (Cowan, 2021) in British culture, might look very different had I experienced more of the exclusions associated with that myself. In Scotland we have had an explicitly nationalist government since 2010, which has also made consistent rhetorical commitments to welcoming immigration and pursuing greater equality in society (Béland and Lecours, 2016). This is not to suggest that Scotland is a social democratic utopia (Frank et al, 2015; Meer, 2015) but only that the things I, personally, associate with nationalism are multiple, and not all malign.

Earlier in the book I reflect on the boldness of this book's title, and since I set my mind on it, it has been apparent how many people it interests and how few people it will please. When I explain the project to people, about half of my audience give the verbal version of an eye roll, envisaging a celebration of NHS heroism which erases all the problems of the NHS in an act of banal nationalism. The other half question the title by telling me bluntly that *they* do not love the NHS, sometimes recounting an awful experience they or a loved one has had, or the impossibility of their current work in the NHS. These responses are, in a sense, further evidence of the NHS's pervasive role in society. My desire to write this book, now, reflects the recurring themes I encountered across research on a range of different topics, and the underlying 'intellectual puzzle' (Mason, 2017) that motivated me to pursue them. Sturdy summarises this neatly, as the tension that 'medicine is concerned with the most intimate aspects of private life. Yet it is also a focus for diverse forms of public organization and action' (Sturdy, 2002). That is, healthcare (its performance, its failures, its controversies) is both resolutely public and intensely private, intimate and personal. Healthcare is thus a landscape for particularly heightened claims-making, and this book explores how these are contested in the UK specifically.

Research design and method

The book combines data and analyses from different studies, and so the following sections explain them individually.

Chapter 3 reports an analysis of crowdfunding pages created by members of the public in the early months of the COVID-19 pandemic. This qualitative analysis was of the written content in 945 JustGiving and GoFundMe pages created to fundraise for the NHSCT COVID-19 Urgent Appeal. With my guidance, Dr Kath Bassett 'captured' the webpages using NVivo between mid-May and mid-June 2020, during the UK's first national lockdown in response to the COVID-19 pandemic. All the JustGiving and GoFundMe pages were available online, within the public domain, and therefore not requiring written consent to analyse. However, to be sensitive to ethical concerns about the potential identifiability of people who wrote such materials (McKee and Porter, 2009; Hlavach and Freivogel, 2011), we have redacted individual names and altered some quotations which seemed potentially identifiable. NVivo was used to code the textual elements of the full population of pages captured. The JustGiving dataset was initially coded by Anna Nonhebel (an undergraduate Medical student studying an intercalated degree in Bioethics, Law and Society) and the Go Fund Me dataset by Dr Chris Möller. There were strong resonances between the inductive codes across the two platforms, and following discussion between all three of us, we agreed a deductive coding framework which was then applied to a combined dataset, with ongoing refinement.

Some of the text of Chapter 3 is adapted from the open access journal article Stewart et al (2022), with the full permission of all co-authors (Anna Nonhebel, Kath Bassett and Chris Möller) and within the licence terms from the publisher Elsevier. Collection of this data was initially funded by my College of Medicine and Vet Medicine Chancellor's Fellowship at the University of Edinburgh, and analysis and writing was conducted under the auspices of my Wellcome Trust Collaborative Award in Humanities and Social Sciences (219901/D/19/Z). Ethical approval was granted by University of Edinburgh's School of Social and Political Science Committee.

Chapter 4 is informed by an auto-ethnographic experience volunteering one afternoon a week for three months in a Royal Voluntary Service café in a Scottish hospital in 2022. Ethical approval for this was granted by University of Strathclyde's School of Social Work and Social Policy Ethics Group, and the research was unfunded. The project was auto-ethnographic (Ellis, Adams and Bochner, 2011), and is therefore focused on my own experiences and reflections as a volunteer. The Royal Voluntary Service, who run the café, and the local volunteering coordinator, were both made aware that I planned to write about my experiences as a volunteer, and I also explained it to my fellow volunteers during our shared shifts. I additionally shared a draft of the chapter with the RVS media team before publication. However customers in the café were not aware of my research, and accordingly I have been circumspect when describing aspects of my volunteering experience which concern interacting with customers, and avoided any identifying details of other people. This element of the research was designed not to stand alone but to ground other data in the chapter on volunteering. Where relevant in Chapter 4, I quote from the extensive reflexive fieldnotes which I wrote immediately after each volunteering shift.

Chapters 4 and 5 also draw on interview data from a series of studies of public roles in the NHS in Scotland, England, Wales and Northern Ireland. All names used are pseudonyms to protect the anonymity of interviewees.

- These include interviews with members of a Public Partnership Forum in Scotland in 2010 for my ESRC-funded PhD studentship (ES/F023405/1). These were semi-structured interviews with members of a forum I had been observing for a few months, with interviews all conducted by me, face-to-face, mostly in Forum members' homes. The data was thematically analysed within the context of my observations of the Forum, and other data sources used in the PhD (a full description of design and methods is available in Stewart, 2012). Ethical approval for that research was granted by University of Edinburgh School of Social and Political Science Ethics Committee.
- Interviews with people volunteering in or campaigning for (or both) local hospitals in Scotland were conducted as part of my Chief Scientist Office Scotland Postdoctoral Fellowship between 2016–18 (grant reference CSO.CF.01). Ethical approval for this research was granted by the University of Edinburgh's Centre for Population Health Sciences Ethics Group. Three qualitative case studies of closure processes included document analysis, interviews with 70 staff, politicians and members of the public and observation at 11 consultation and community meetings. Interviews were conducted by me, in person, in a mixture of venues including interviewee's homes, cafes and meeting spaces. This data was analysed using a grounded theory approach, along with fieldnotes and extensive documentary sources from the cases. A full description of design and methods is available in the methodological appendix for Stewart (2019). An additional case study for this project was undertaken by Dr Kathy Dodworth in 2018, and these 10 interviews with campaigners were thematically analysed in NVivo. The design and methods for this final case study is reported in Dodworth and Stewart (2022). Each quote is accompanied by a pseudonym, the study identifier (CSO), and the case study number (1–4).
- Further interviews with hospital campaigners in England, Wales and Northern Ireland were conducted as part of a Health Foundation Policy Challenge Fund grant (reference 7607) held with Professors Scott Greer and Peter D. Donnelly between 2016 and 2018. This grant involved eight case studies of hospital change processes, two in each of England, Wales, Northern Ireland and Scotland. Eight semi-structured interviews with hospital campaigners were conducted by myself or Dr Angelo Ercia, and thematically analysed together using NVivo software. Each quote is accompanied by a pseudonym, the funder abbreviation (HF), and the country (England, Northern Ireland, Scotland or Wales). Full

details of the design and methods for this study are available in Stewart et al (2020).

Some of the text in Chapter 5 is adapted from a co-authored chapter in an open access edited collection (Stewart, Dodworth and Erica, 2022), with kind agreement from my co-authors Kathy Dodworth, Angelo Ercia, and the publisher Manchester University Press.

Chapter 5 also draws on new, unfunded analysis of online campaign materials from two national campaigns: Keep our NHS Public, and Your NHS Needs You. Using NCapture for NVivo, I captured the webpages of each campaign as at 10 August 2022. I also watched the 45 Your NHS Needs You videos of 476 'celebrities' explaining their support for the campaign (as listed in Table A.1), and either downloaded the auto-generated YouTube transcripts, or transcribed my own where these were not available. These transcripts were included in a thematic analysis of all the web materials.

Chapter 6 reports a new analysis of patient narratives submitted to Care Opinion website. Ethical advice was sought from University of Strathclyde School of Social Work & Social Policy, who confirmed that as the data is in the public domain, formal ethical approval was not required. Care Opinion generously gave me a free subscription to their website to enable the research, which allowed me to easily search and then extract to Excel, the text of stories. When I conducted this research in 2022, Care Opinion had over 500,000 total stories available in their database, dating back 16 years. I explored various options for reducing the number of stories to a manageable corpus for analysis. The search facility is designed for organisations within the NHS to identify stories of care they have delivered. There are options for text searching and the use of wild cards, although given the breadth of my interest in how 'the NHS' is referenced within narratives of care, these were of limited use, often catching the names of organisations (for example, NHS 24 or NHS Lothian). In the end I followed the following parameters for the search:

- I focused only on stories of emergency medicine, rather than a specific specialism. Chapter 6 discusses this limitation further, but my rationale was, first, because emergency medicine operates as a gateway to NHS care, and the other obvious alternative (primary care) has a more complex contractual relationship to the NHS. Second, emergency medicine is often where system problems become particularly visible to a wider audience: both in terms of waiting times and because of the unscheduled nature of emergency care (Hillman, 2014; Grant and Hoyle, 2017).
- I selected two one-year time periods (2019 and 2021). These snapshots allow me to explore how the NHS was discussed before and during the COVID-19 pandemics, while still allowing shifts in discussion across the

Table A.1: List of celebrity videos for Your NHS Needs You analysed in Chapter 5

Celebrity videos for Your NHS Needs You campaign
Adam Kay
Angela Barnes
Barry Gardiner MP
Bell Ribiero-Addy MP
Ben Bailey-Smith
Brian Eno
Caroline Lucas
Charlotte Church
Dave Ward
David Tennant
Dr Julia Patterson
Emma Kennedy
Frankie Boyle
George Monbiot
Graeme Garden MP
Jen Brister
Jeremy Corbyn MP
Jessica Fostokew
Jo Brand
Joe Lycett
Johnny Vegas
Jonathan Ross
Julie Hemondhalgh
Kiri Protchard-McLean
Lee Ridley
Lemn Sissay
Marcus Brigstocke and Rachel Parris
Margaret Greenwood MP
Michael Rosen
Peter Stefanovic
Rebecca Long-Bailey MP
Richard Burgon MP
Robin Ince
Romesh Ranganathan

Table A.1: List of celebrity videos for Your NHS Needs You analysed in Chapter 5 (continued)

Celebrity videos for Your NHS Needs You campaign
Rosie Jones
Russell Brand
Saffron Burrows
Samuel West
Shami Chakrabati
Shappi Khorsandi
Stephen Fry
Steve Coogan
Suzi Ruffell
Vicky McClure
Yanis Varoufakis

calendar year (for example, reflecting longstanding 'winter pressures' in emergency medicine) to be apparent.
- I only included stories added to the database via Care Opinion itself. Some stories are also added via the www.nhs.uk website in England, but there are various differences with this interface which make inclusion unhelpful for our purposes, including that stories are not assigned a 'criticality' rating (Care Opinion, 2022b).

I removed any duplicate stories, and manually 'cleaned' the data to exclude stories where the mention of the NHS was only due to the name of a specific organisation. I uploaded the data to NVivo, and spent some time familiarising myself with the data. Far from a dry technical process, reading these narratives is absorbing and often upsetting, given the experiences described within. I developed a thematic analysis coding framework based on this reading. Before coding the dataset, I discussed the coding framework with my colleague Fadhila Mazanderani, who has interviewed people about their experiences of submitting feedback online (Mazanderani et al, 2021), and her feedback shaped the analysis.

References

Acheson, N., Crawford, L., Grotz, J., Hardill, I., Hayward, D., Hogg, E. et al (2022). *Mobilising the Voluntary Sector: Critical Reflections from Across the Four UK Nations – COVID-19 and the Voluntary and Community Sector in the UK* (pp 17–29). Bristol: Policy Press. Retrieved from https://bristoluniversityp ressdigital.com/display/book/9781447365532/ch002.xml

Addley, E. (2020, 28 May). Clap for our Carers: The Very Un-British Ritual that United the Nation. *The Guardian*. Retrieved from www.theguardian. com/society/2020/may/28/clap-for-our-carers-the-very-unbritish-rit ual-that-united-the-nation

Ahmed, S. (2010). *The Promise of Happiness*. Durham, NC: Duke University Press. Retrieved from https://doi.org/10.1515/9780822392781

Appleby, J., Harrison, A. and Devlin, N. (2003). *What Is the Real Cost of More Patient Choice?* London: King's Fund. Retrieved from www.kings fund.org.uk/sites/default/files/field/field_publication_file/what-is-real- cost-more-patient-choice-john-appleby-tony-harrison-nancy-devlin- kings-fund-1-june-2003.pdf

Arnold-Forster, A. (2022, 9 March). Carbolic Soap Operas. Retrieved from www.lrb.co.uk/blog/2022/march/carbolic-soap-operas

Arnold-Forster, A. and Gainty, C. (2021). To Save the NHS We Need to Stop Loving It. *Renewal*, 29(4), 9.

Bailey, S. and West, M. (2021, 14 June). Naming the Issue: Chronic Excessive Workload in the NHS. Retrieved from www.kingsfund.org.uk/blog/2021/ 06/naming-issue-chronic-excessive-workload-nhs

Baines, R., Underwood, F., O'Keeffe, K., Saunders, J. and Jones, R. B. (2021). Implementing Online Patient Feedback in a 'Special Measures' Acute Hospital: A Case Study Using Normalisation Process Theory. *Digital Health*, 7. Retrieved from https://doi.org/10.1177/2055207621 1005962

Bambra, C. (2005a). Cash Versus Services: 'Worlds of Welfare' and the Decommodification of Cash Benefits and Health Care Services. *Journal of Social Policy*, 34(2), 195–213. Retrieved from https://doi.org/10.1017/ S0047279404008542

Bambra, C. (2005b). Worlds of Welfare and the Health Care Discrepancy. *Social Policy and Society*, 4(1), 31–41. Retrieved from https://doi.org/ 10.1017/S1474746404002143

Bambra, C., Lynch, J. and Smith, K. E. (2021). *The Unequal Pandemic: COVID- 19 and Health Inequalities*. Bristol: Policy Press.

Bandola-Gill, J., Grek, S. and Tichenor, M. (2022). The Sustainable Development Goals as Epistemic Infrastructures. In J. Bandola-Gill, S. Grek and M. Tichenor (Eds), *Governing the Sustainable Development Goals: Quantification in Global Public Policy* (pp 1–17). Cham: Springer International Publishing. Retrieved from https://doi.org/10.1007/978-3-031-03938-6_1

Barcelos, C. A. (2020). Go Fund Inequality: The Politics of Crowdfunding Transgender Medical Care. *Critical Public Health*, 30(3), 330–339. Retrieved from https://doi.org/10.1080/09581596.2019.1575947

Barnes, B. (1993). Power. In R. Bellamy (Ed), *Theories and Concepts of Politics: An Introduction* (pp 197–219). Manchester: Manchester University Press.

Barratt, H., Harrison, D. A., Fulop, N. J. and Raine, R. (2015). Factors that Influence the Way Communities Respond to Proposals for Major Changes to Local Emergency Services: A Qualitative Study. *PLoS ONE*, 10(3). Retrieved from https://doi.org/10.1371/journal.pone.0120766

Barrett, D. (2021). MPs Praise Mail's 'Brilliant' Helpforce in Volunteer Drive. *The Daily Mail*. Retrieved from www.dailymail.co.uk/news/article-10134519/Mail-campaign-gets-thumbs-report-proposes-raft-measures-Britons-volunteering.html

BBC News Online. (2022, 1 December). My Mum's 40-hour Wait to Get to A&E with Hip Break. *BBC News*. Retrieved from www.bbc.com/news/health-63808516

Béland, D. and Lecours, A. (2005). The Politics of Territorial Solidarity: Nationalism and Social Policy Reform in Canada, the United Kingdom, and Belgium. *Comparative Political Studies*, 38(6), 676–703. Retrieved from https://doi.org/10.1177/0010414005275600

Béland, D. and Lecours, A. (2016). The 2014 Scottish Referendum and the Nationalism-Social Policy Nexus. *Canadian Political Science Review*, 10(1), 1–30.

Berry, E., Skea, Z. C., Campbell, M. K. and Locock, L. (2022). 'Using Humanity to Change Systems' – Understanding the Work of Online Feedback Moderation: A Case Study of Care Opinion Scotland. *Digital Health*, 8, 20552076211074490. Retrieved from https://doi.org/10.1177/20552076211074489

Berwick, D. M. (2008). A Transatlantic Review of the NHS at 60. *British Medical Journal*, 337, a838. Retrieved from https://doi.org/10.1136/bmj.a838

Bevan, A. (2010). *In Place of Fear*. Whitefish, MT: Kessinger Publishing.

Bevan, G., Karanikolos, M., Exley, J., Nolte, E., Connolly, S. and Mays, N. (2014). *The Four Health Systems of the United Kingdom: How Do They Compare?* London: The Health Foundation; Nuffield Trust. Retrieved from www.nuffieldtrust.org.uk/sites/files/nuffield/revised_4_countries_report.pdf

Bhambra, G. K. (2022a). Relations of Extraction, Relations of Redistribution: Empire, Nation, and the Construction of the British Welfare State. *The British Journal of Sociology*, 73(1), 4–15. Retrieved from https://doi.org/10.1111/1468-4446.12896

Bhambra, G. K. (2022b). Webs of Reciprocity: Colonial Taxation and the Need for Reparations. *The British Journal of Sociology*, 73(1), 73–77. Retrieved from https://doi.org/10.1111/1468-4446.12908

Bird, S. and Boyle, D. (2014). *Give and Take: How Timebanking is Transforming Healthcare*. Stroud: Timebanking UK.

Bivins, R. (2015). *Contagious Communities: Medicine, Migration, and the NHS in Post-war Britain*. Oxford: Oxford University Press.

Bivins, R. (2020). Commentary: Serving the Nation, Serving the People: Echoes of War in the Early NHS. *Medical Humanities*, 46(2), 154–156. Retrieved from https://doi.org/10.1136/medhum-2019-011760

Black Equity Organisation and Clearview Research. (2022). *Systemic Change Required*. UK: Black Equity Organisation. Retrieved from https://black equityorg.com/wp-content/uploads/2022/09/Systemic-change-requi red-V10.pdf

Bochel, H. and Defty, A. (2010). Safe as Houses? Conservative Social Policy, Public Opinion and Parliament. *The Political Quarterly*, 81(1), 74–84. Retrieved from https://doi.org/10.1111/j.1467-923X.2009.02064.x

Bochel, H. and Powell, M. (2018). Whatever Happened to Compassionate Conservatism Under the Coalition Government? *British Politics*, 13(2), 146–170. Retrieved from https://doi.org/10.1057/s41293-016-0028-2

Bonvin, J.-M. and Laruffa, F. (2022). Towards a Capability-Oriented Eco-Social Policy: Elements of a Normative Framework. *Social Policy and Society*, 21(3), 484–495. Retrieved from https://doi.org/10.1017/S14747 46421000798

Borland, S. (2018, 2 December). More than 7,000 People Sign Up to Daily Mail Christmas NHS Campaign. *Mail Online*. Retrieved from www.dailym ail.co.uk/news/article-6452663/More-7-000-volunteers-sign-NHS-48-hours-Daily-Mail-launches-campaign.html

Bowles, J., Clifford, D. and Mohan, J. (2023). The Place of Charity in a Public Health Service: Inequality and Persistence in Charitable Support for NHS Trusts in England. *Social Science & Medicine*, 322. Retrieved from https://doi.org/10.1016/j.socscimed.2023.115805

Bradby, H. (2012). *Medicine, Health and Society*. Thousand Oaks, CA: SAGE.

Bradby, H., Lindenmeyer, A., Phillimore, J., Padilla, B. and Brand, T. (2020). 'If There Were Doctors Who Could Understand Our Problems, I Would Already Be Better': Dissatisfactory Health Care and Marginalisation in Superdiverse Neighbourhoods. *Sociology of Health & Illness*, 42(4), 739–757. Retrieved from https://doi.org/10.1111/1467-9566.13061

Bradley, P., Wilson, A., Buss, P., Harrhy, S., Laing, H., Shortland, G. and van Woerden, H. (2014). *Achieving Prudent Healthcare in NHS Wales*. Cardiff: Public Health Wales. Retrieved from https://pure.uhi.ac.uk/files/1921669/Achieving_prudent_healthcare_in_NHS_Wales_paper_Revised _version_FINAL_.pdf

Brennan, N., Langdon, N., Bryce, M., Gale, T., Knapton, A., Burns, L. and Humphries, N. (2021). *Drivers of International Migration of Doctors to and from the United Kingdom* (No. ITT GMC996). Retrieved from Plymouth: CAMERA; Peninsula Medical School.

Brewis, G. (2013). *Towards a New Understanding of Volunteering in England before 1960?* London: Institute for Volunteering. Retrieved from https://discovery.ucl.ac.uk/id/eprint/1560893/1/IVR_working_paper_two_history_of_volunteering.pdf

Brindle, D. (2020, 6 May). Ellie Orton: 'The £92m We've Raised for the NHS Will Never Replace State Funding'. *The Guardian*. Retrieved from https://www.theguardian.com/society/2020/may/06/ellie-orton-92m-nhs-state-funding-captain-tom

Britnell, M. (2015). *In Search of the Perfect Health System*. London: Bloomsbury Publishing.

Brookes, G., McEnery, T., McGlashan, M., Smith, G. and Wilkinson, M. (2022). Narrative Evaluation in Patient Feedback: A Study of Online Comments about UK Healthcare Services. *Narrative Inquiry*, 32(1), 9–35. Retrieved from https://doi.org/10.1075/ni.20098.bro

Brown, L. D. (2015). Review of Rudolf Klein, The New Politics of the NHS: From Creation to Reinvention. *Health Economics, Policy and Law*, 10(2), 237–240. Retrieved from https://doi.org/10.1017/S1744133114000309

Brown, P. and Zavestoski, S. (2004). Social Movements in Health: An Introduction. *Sociology of Health & Illness*, 26(6), 679–694. Retrieved from https://doi.org/10.1111/j.0141-9889.2004.00413.x

Broyard, A. (1992). *Intoxicated by My Illness: And Other Writings on Life and Death*. New York: Clarkson Potter. Retrieved from https://repository.library.georgetown.edu/handle/10822/851737

Bueger, C. (2015). Making Things Known: Epistemic Practices, the United Nations, and the Translation of Piracy. *International Political Sociology*, 9(1), 1–18. Retrieved from https://doi.org/10.1111/ips.12073

Burlacu, D. and Roescu, A. (2021). Public Opinion on Healthcare. In E. M. Immergut, K. M. Anderson, C. Devitt and T. Popic (Eds), *Health Politics in Europe* (pp 49–70). Oxford: Oxford University Press. Retrieved from https://doi.org/10.1093/oso/9780198860525.003.0003

Buzelli, L., Cameron, G., Gardner, T., Williamson, S. and Alderwick, H. (2022). *Public Perceptions of Health and Social Care: What the New Government Should Know – The Health Foundation*. London: The Health Foundation. Retrieved from https://www.health.org.uk/publications/reports/public-perceptions-of-health-and-social-care-what-government-should-know

Care Opinion. (2022a). How is Care Opinion funded? Retrieved from https://www.careopinion.org.uk/info/funding

Care Opinion. (2022b). Working with nhs.uk. Retrieved from https://www.careopinion.org.uk/info/nhs-uk

Care Quality Commission. (2022). NHS Patient Survey Programme. Retrieved from https://www.cqc.org.uk/publications/surveys

Carpenter, D. (2012). Is Health Politics Different? *Annual Review of Political Science*, 15(1), 287–311. Retrieved from https://doi.org/10.1146/annurev-polisci-050409-113009

Carrington, O. (2021). NHS Charities Financial Comparison Dashboard 2020 – Part 2. Retrieved from https://public.tableau.com/app/profile/oliver.carrington2982/viz/NHScharitiesfinancialcomparisondashboard2020/Page2-income#1

Carter, P. and Martin, G. (2018). Engagement of Patients and the Public in NHS Sustainability and Transformation: An Ethnographic Study. *Critical Social Policy*, 38(4). Retrieved from https://doi.org/10.1177/0261018317749387

Centre for Health and the Public Interest. (2022). *Briefing: The Bet Against the NHS – How Likely Is a Two-tier Healthcare System in the UK?* London: Centre for Health and the Public Interest. Retrieved from https://chpi.org.uk/wp-content/uploads/2022/10/The-Bet-Against-the-NHS-October-2022.pdf

Charlesworth, A. and Bloor, K. (2018). 70 Years of NHS Funding: How Do We Know How Much Is Enough? *BMJ*, 361, k2373. Retrieved from https://doi.org/10.1136/bmj.k2373

Cherry, S. (2000). Hospital Saturday, Workplace Collections and Issues in Late Nineteenth-century Hospital Funding. *Medical History*, 44(4), 461–488. Retrieved from https://doi.org/10.1017/S0025727300067089

Clarke, J. and Newman, J. (2007). What's in a Name? *Cultural Studies*, 21(4–5), 738–757. Retrieved from https://doi.org/10.1080/09502380701279051

Clarke, J., Newman, J., Smith, N., Vidler, E. and Westmarland, L. (2007). *Creating Citizen-consumers: Changing Publics & Changing Public Services*. Thousand Oaks, CA: SAGE.

Coates, S. (2021). Population Estimates by Ethnic Group and Religion, England and Wales – Office for National Statistics. Retrieved from https://www.ons.gov.uk/peoplepopulationandcommunity/populationandmigration/populationestimates/articles/populationestimatesbyethnicgroupandreligionenglandandwales/2019

Cohen, N., Mizrahi, S. and Vigoda-Gadot, E. (2022). Alternative Provision of Public Health Care: The Role of Citizens' Satisfaction with Public Services and the Social Responsibility of Government. *Health Economics, Policy and Law*, 17(2), 121–140. Retrieved from https://doi.org/10.1017/S1744133120000201

Collins, M. E., Rum, S. A. and Sugarman, J. (2018). Navigating the Ethical Boundaries of Grateful Patient Fundraising. *JAMA*, 320(10), 975–976. Retrieved from https://doi.org/10.1001/jama.2018.11655

Collins, M. E., Rum, S., Wheeler, J., Antman, K., Brem, H., Carrese, J. et al (2018). Ethical Issues and Recommendations in Grateful Patient Fundraising and Philanthropy. *Academic Medicine*, 93(11), 1631–1637. Retrieved from https://doi.org/10.1097/ACM.0000000000002365

Commission on Social Security. (2022). The Plan. Retrieved from https://www.commissiononsocialsecurity.org

Cooper, K. and Burchardt, T. (2022). How Divided is the Attitudinal Context for Policymaking? Changes in Public Attitudes to the Welfare State, Inequality and Immigration Over Two Decades in Britain. *Social Policy & Administration*, 56(1), 1–18. Retrieved from https://doi.org/10.1111/spol.12739

Cowan, H. (2020). *How I Fell Out of Love with the NHS: An Ethnography of Hip Replacements and Healthcare Assemblages in the UK* (Doctoral thesis). London School of Hygiene & Tropical Medicine. Retrieved from https://doi.org/10.17037/PUBS.04658095

Cowan, H. (2021). Taking the National(ism) out of the National Health Service: Re-locating Agency to amongst Ourselves. *Critical Public Health*, 31(2), 134–143. Retrieved from https://doi.org/10.1080/09581596.2020.1836328

Cox, C. L. (2020). 'Healthcare Heroes': Problems with Media Focus on Heroism from Healthcare Workers During the COVID-19 Pandemic. *Journal of Medical Ethics*, 46(8), 510–513. Retrieved from https://doi.org/10.1136/medethics-2020-106398

Crane, J. (2019). 'Save Our NHS': Activism, Information-based Expertise and the 'New Times' of the 1980s. *Contemporary British History*, 33(1), 52–74. Retrieved from https://doi.org/10.1080/13619462.2018.1525299

Crane, J. (2022). 'Loving' the National Health Service: Social Surveys and Activist Feelings. In J. Crane and J. Hand (Eds), *Posters, Protests and Prescriptions: Cultural Histories of the National Health Service* (pp 79–102). Manchester: Manchester University Press. Retrieved from https://www.manchesteropenhive.com/view/9781526163479/9781526163479.00012.xml

Crane, J. and Hand, J. (Eds). (2022). *Posters, Protests, and Prescriptions: Cultural Histories of the National Health Service in Britain*. Manchester: Manchester University Press.

Cresswell, R. (2020). The 'British Red Cross Still Exists', 1947–74: Finding a Role After the Second World War. In N. Wylie, M. Oppenheimer and J. Crossland (Eds), *The Red Cross Movement* (pp 148–163). Manchester: Manchester University Press. Retrieved from https://manchesteruniversitypress.co.uk/shsconference2021/9781526133519/

Cribb, A. (2018). *Healthcare in Transition: Understanding Key Ideas and Tensions in Contemporary Health Policy*. Bristol: Policy Press.

Curtice, J. (2016). *The Benefits of Random Sampling: Lessons from the 2015 General Election*. London: NatCen. Retrieved from https://www.bsa.nat cen.ac.uk/media/39018/random-sampling.pdf

Dallinger, U. (2022). On the Ambivalence of Preferences for Income Redistribution: A Research Note. *Journal of European Social Policy*, 32(2). Retrieved from https://doi.org/10.1177/09589287211066469

Dalton, J., Chambers, D., Harden, M., Street, A., Parker, G. and Eastwood, A. (2016). Service User Engagement in Health Service Reconfiguration: A Rapid Evidence Synthesis. *Journal of Health Services Research & Policy*, 21(3), 195–205. Retrieved from https://doi.org/10.1177/1355819615623305

Daly, M. and Lewis, J. (2000). The Concept of Social Care and the Analysis of Contemporary Welfare States. *The British Journal of Sociology*, 51(2), 281–298. Retrieved from https://doi.org/10.1111/j.1468-4446.2000.00281.x

Darlington-Pollock, F. (2022). *Disease*. Newcastle-upon-Tyne: Agenda Publishing.

Davidson, D., Paine, A. E., Glasby, J., Williams, I., Tucker, H., Crilly, T. et al (2019). Analysis of the Profile, Characteristics, Patient Experience and Community Value of Community Hospitals: A Multimethod Study. *Health Services and Delivery Research*, 7. Retrieved from https://doi.org/10.3310/hsdr07010

Davies, C. (2003). Some of Our Concepts Are Missing: Reflections on the Absence of a Sociology of Organisations in Sociology of Health and Illness. *Sociology of Health & Illness*, 25(3), 172–190.

Day, G., Robert, G., Leedham-Green, K. and Rafferty, A. M. (2022). An Outbreak of Appreciation: A Discursive Analysis of Tweets of Gratitude Expressed to the National Health Service at the Outset of the COVID-19 Pandemic. *Health Expectations*, 25(1), 149–162. Retrieved from https://doi.org/10.1111/hex.13359

De Cleen, B., Moffitt, B., Panayotu, P. and Stavrakakis, Y. (2020). The Potentials and Difficulties of Transnational Populism: The Case of the Democracy in Europe Movement 2025 (DiEM25). *Political Studies*, 68(1), 146–166. Retrieved from https://doi.org/10.1177/0032321719847576

de Vries, R., Baumberg Geiger, B., Scullion, L., Summers, K., Edmiston, D., Ingold, J. et al (2020). *Solidarity in a Crisis? Trends in Attitudes to Benefits During COVID-19* (No. 978-1-912337-52-1). Manchester: Welfare at a (Social) Distance. Retrieved from https://www.distantwelfare.co.uk/attitudes

Dean, J. (2020). *The Good Glow: Charity and the Symbolic Power of Doing Good*. Bristol: Policy Press.

Dean, R., Boswell, J. and Smith, G. (2019). Designing Democratic Innovations as Deliberative Systems: The Ambitious Case of NHS Citizen. *Political Studies*, 68(3). Retrieved from https://doi.org/10.1177/00323 21719866002

Della Porta, D. (2013). Repertoires of Contention. In D. Snow, D. Della Porta, D. McAdam and B. Klandermans (Eds), *The Wiley-Blackwell Encyclopedia of Social and Political Movements* (pp 1–3). Blackwell Publishing Ltd. Retrieved from http://onlinelibrary.wiley.com/doi/10.1002/978047 0674871.wbespm178/abstract

Department of Health. (2002). *Learning from Bristol: The Department of Health's Response to the Report of the Public Inquiry into Children's Heart Surgery at the Bristol Royal Infirmary 1984–1995.* London: Stationery Office.

Department of Health. (2011). *Opportunities for Volunteering: The Legacy Report.* London: Department of Health.

Djellouli, N., Jones, L., Barratt, H., Ramsay, A. I. G., Towndrow, S. and Oliver, S. (2019). Involving the Public in Decision-making About Large-scale Changes to Health Services: A Scoping Review. *Health Policy*, 123(7), 635–645. Retrieved from https://doi.org/10.1016/j.healthpol.2019.05.006

Dodworth, K. and Stewart, E. (2022). Legitimating Complementary Therapies in the NHS: Campaigning, Care and Epistemic Labour. *Health*, 26(2), 244–262. Retrieved from https://doi.org/10.1177/1363459320931916

Dolan, P., Krekel, C., Shreedhar, G., Lee, H., Marshall, C. and Smith, A. (2021). *Happy to Help: The Welfare Effects of a Nationwide Micro-Volunteering Programme* (Discussion paper No. 2042–2695). London: Centre for Economic Performance. Retrieved from https://www.ssrn.com/abstract=3865456

Duffy, B. (2021). *The NHS and Public Health: Perceptions vs Reality.* London: The Health Foundation; King's College London Policy Institute. Retrieved from https://www.kcl.ac.uk/policy-institute/assets/nhs-and-public-health-perceptions-vs-reality.pdf

Duncan, C. (1998). The Elusive Nature of NHS Crises. *The Political Quarterly*, 69(4), 432–440. Retrieved from https://doi.org/10.1111/1467-923X.00179

Eakin, J. M. and Mykhalovskiy, E. (2003). Reframing the Evaluation of Qualitative Health Research: Reflections on a Review of Appraisal Guidelines in the Health Sciences. *Journal of Evaluation in Clinical Practice*, 9(2), 187–194. Retrieved from https://doi.org/10.1046/j.1365-2753.2003.00392.x

Edwards, C., Staniszewska, S. and Crichton, N. (2004). Investigation of the Ways in Which Patients' Reports of Their Satisfaction with Healthcare Are Constructed. *Sociology of Health & Illness*, 26(2), 159–183. Retrieved from https://doi.org/10.1111/j.1467-9566.2004.00385.x

Edwards, N. (2022a, 19 October). Myth #1: We Already Spend Too Much on Health: And Despite This Our Outcomes Are Poor. Retrieved from https://www.nuffieldtrust.org.uk/news-item/myth-1-we-already-spend-too-much-on-health-and-our-outcomes-are-poor

Edwards, N. (2022b, 24 October). Myth #2: The NHS is a 'Sacred Cow' that Evades Reform, and its Exceptionalism Is its Weakness. Retrieved from https://www.nuffieldtrust.org.uk/news-item/myth-2-the-nhs-is-a-sacred-cow-that-evades-reform-and-its-exceptionalism-is-its-weakness

Eliasoph, N. (1998). *Avoiding Politics: How Americans Produce Apathy in Everyday Life*. New York: Cambridge University Press.

Elkind, A. (1998). Using Metaphor to Read the Organisation of the NHS. *Social Science & Medicine*, 47(11), 1715–1727. Retrieved from https://doi.org/10.1016/S0277-9536(98)00251-2

Ellis, C., Adams, T. E. and Bochner, A. P. (2011). Autoethnography: An Overview. *Forum Qualitative Sozialforschung/Forum: Qualitative Social Research*, 12(1). Retrieved from https://doi.org/10.17169/fqs-12.1.1589

Epstein, S. (2016). The Politics of Health Mobilization in the United States: The Promise and Pitfalls of 'Disease Constituencies'. *Social Science & Medicine*, 165, 246–254. Retrieved from https://doi.org/10.1016/j.socscimed.2016.01.048

Erikainen, S. and Stewart, E. (2020). Credibility Contests: Media Debates on Do-It-Yourself Coronavirus Responses and the Role of Citizens in Health Crises. *Frontiers in Sociology*, 0. Retrieved from https://doi.org/10.3389/fsoc.2020.592666

Esping-Andersen, G. (2013). *The Three Worlds of Welfare Capitalism*. Hoboken, NJ: John Wiley & Sons.

Ewbank, L., Thompson, J., McKenna, H., Anandaciva, S. and Ward, D. (2021). NHS Hospital Bed Numbers: Past, Present and Future. Retrieved from https://www.kingsfund.org.uk/publications/nhs-hospital-bed-numbers

Ewbank, L., Wellings, D., Wenzel, L., Burkitt, R., Duxbury, K., Gregory, F. and Hall, S. (2018). *The Public and the NHS: What's the Deal?* London: King's Fund. Retrieved from https://www.kingsfund.org.uk/publications/public-and-nhs-whats-the-deal

Farnsworth, K. (2021). Retrenched, Reconfigured and Broken: The British Welfare State after a Decade of Austerity. *Social Policy and Society*, 20(1), 77–96. Retrieved from https://doi.org/10.1017/S1474746420000524

Feeley, D. (2008, February). Refreshed Strategy for Volunteering in the NHS in Scotland. CEL. Retrieved from https://www.sehd.scot.nhs.uk/mels/CEL2008_10.pdf

Ferreira, M. R., Proença, T. and Proença, J. F. (2012). Motivation among Hospital Volunteers: An Empirical Analysis in Portugal. *International Review on Public and Nonprofit Marketing*, 9(2), 137–152. Retrieved from https://doi.org/10.1007/s12208-012-0083-3

Filc, D. (2014). The Role of Civil Society in Health Care Reforms: An Arena for Hegemonic Struggles. *Social Science & Medicine*, 123, 168–173. Retrieved from https://doi.org/10.1016/j.socscimed.2014.07.030

Firth, A. (2013). Volunteering and Managing Change in the Health Sector. *Perspectives in Public Health*, 133(5), 240.

Fitzgerald, D., Hinterberger, A., Narayan, J. and Williams, R. (2020). Brexit as Heredity Redux: Imperialism, Biomedicine and the NHS in Britain. *The Sociological Review*, 68(6), 1161–1178.

Fortier, A.-M. (2016). Afterword: Acts of Affective Citizenship? Possibilities and Limitations. *Citizenship Studies*, 20(8), 1038–1044. Retrieved from https://doi.org/10.1080/13621025.2016.1229190

Foucault, M. (2014). The Politics of Health in the Eighteenth Century. *Foucault Studies*, 18, 113–127.

Francis, G. (2015). *Adventures in Human Being.* London: Profile Books.

Francis-Devine, B., Powell, A. and Clark, H. (2021). *Coronavirus Job Retention Scheme: statistics* (Commons Library Research Briefing No. 9152). London: The House of Commons Library. Retrieved from https://researchbriefings.files.parliament.uk/documents/CBP-9152/CBP-9152.pdf

Frank, J., Bromley, C., Doi, L., Estrade, M., Jepson, R., McAteer, J. et al (2015). Seven Key Investments for Health Equity Across the Lifecourse: Scotland versus the Rest of the UK. *Social Science & Medicine*, 140, 136–146. Retrieved from https://doi.org/10.1016/j.socscimed.2015.07.007

Freeman, R. (2008). A National Health Service, By Comparison. *Social History of Medicine*, 21(3), 503–520. Retrieved from https://doi.org/10.1093/shm/hkn065

Freeman, R. and Frisina, L. (2010). Health Care Systems and the Problem of Classification. *Journal of Comparative Policy Analysis: Research and Practice*, 12(1–2), 163–178. Retrieved from https://doi.org/10.1080/13876980903076278

Fulop, N. J., Walters, R., Perri 6 and Spurgeon, P. (2012). Implementing Changes to Hospital Services: Factors Influencing the Process and 'Results' of Reconfiguration. *Health Policy*, 104(2), 128–135. Retrieved from https://doi.org/10.1016/j.healthpol.2011.05.015

Galea, A., Naylor, C., Buck, D. and Weaks, L. (2013). *Volunteering in Acute Trusts in England: Understanding the Scale and Impact.* London: King's Fund. Retrieved from: https://www.kingsfund.org.uk/sites/default/files/field/field_publication_file/volunteering-in-acute-trusts-in-england-kingsfund-nov13.pdf

Ganguli-Mitra, A., Young, I., Engelmann, L., Harper, I., McCormack, D., Marsland, R. et al (2020, 26 May). Segmenting Communities as Public Health Strategy: A View from the Social Sciences and Humanities. [Version 1; peer review: 2 approved.] *Wellcome Open Research.* Retrieved from https://doi.org/10.12688/wellcomeopenres.15975.1

Garthwaite, K. (2016). Stigma, Shame and 'People Like Us': An Ethnographic Study of Foodbank Use in the UK. *Journal of Poverty and Social Justice*, 24(3), 277–289. Retrieved from https://doi.org/10.1332/175982716X1472195 4314922

Geiger, S. (2021). *Healthcare Activism, Marketization, and the Collective Good.* Oxford: Oxford University Press. Retrieved from https://doi.org/10.1093/oso/9780198865223.003.0001

Gerada, C. (2021). Clare Gerada: Happy birthday, NHS. *BMJ*, 374, n1917. Retrieved from https://doi.org/10.1136/bmj.n1917

Gevers, J., Gelissen, J., Arts, W. and Muffels, R. (2000). Public Health Care in the Balance: Exploring Popular Support for Health Care Systems in the European Union. *International Journal of Social Welfare*, 9(4), 301–321. Retrieved from https://doi.org/10.1111/1468-2397.00141

Gilbert, D. (2014). We Are All Patients. Yes And No. Retrieved from https://www.inhealthassociates.co.uk/uncategorized/we-are-all-patients-yes-and-no-2/

Gilbert, D. (2019). *The Patient Revolution: How We Can Heal the Healthcare System.* Philadelphia, PA: Jessica Kingsley Publishers.

Gillespie, A. and Reader, T. W. (2022). Online Patient Feedback as a Safety Valve: An Automated Language Analysis of Unnoticed and Unresolved Safety Incidents. *Risk Analysis*, Early View. Retrieved from https://doi.org/10.1111/risa.14002

Glynos, J. and Speed, E. (2012). Varieties of Co-production in Public Services: Time Banks in a UK Health Policy Context. *Critical Policy Studies*, 6(4), 402–433.

Gonzales, A. L., Kwon, E. Y., Lynch, T. and Fritz, N. (2018). 'Better Everyone Should Know Our Business Than We Lose Our House': Costs and Benefits of Medical Crowdfunding for Support, Privacy, and Identity. *New Media & Society*, 20(2), 641–658. Retrieved from https://doi.org/10.1177/1461444816667723

Gorsky, M. (2008). The British National Health Service 1948–2008: A Review of the Historiography. *Social History of Medicine*, 21(3), 437–460. Retrieved from https://doi.org/10.1093/shm/hkn064

Gorsky, M. (2015). 'Voluntarism' in English Health and Welfare: Visions of History. In S. Lucey and V. Crossman (Eds), *Health Care, Voluntarism and Regionalism in Ireland and Britain 1850–1950* (pp 31–60). London: University of London Press.

Gorsky, M., Mohan, J. and Willis, T. (2005). From Hospital Contributory Schemes to Health Cash Plans: The Mutual Idea in British Health Care After 1948. *Journal of Social Policy*, 34(3), 447–467.

Gorsky, M. and Sheard, S. (2006). *Financing Medicine: The British Experience Since 1750.* Abingdon: Routledge.

Gosling, G. C. (2017). *Payment and Philanthropy in British Healthcare, 1918–48.* Manchester: Manchester University Press. Retrieved from http://www.ncbi.nlm.nih.gov/books/NBK441616/

Grant, A. and Hoyle, L. (2017). Print Media Representations of UK Accident and Emergency Treatment Targets: Winter 2014–2015. *Journal of Clinical Nursing*, 26(23–24), 4425–4435. Retrieved from https://doi.org/10.1111/jocn.13772

Gray, M. and Barford, A. (2018). The Depths of the Cuts: The Uneven Geography of Local Government Austerity. *Cambridge Journal of Regions, Economy and Society*, 11(3), 541–563. Retrieved from https://doi.org/10.1093/cjres/rsy019

Green, J. and Hobolt, S. B. (2008). Owning the Issue Agenda: Party Strategies and Vote Choices in British Elections. *Electoral Studies*, 27(3), 460–476. Retrieved from https://doi.org/10.1016/j.electstud.2008.02.003

Greener, I. (2022). *Welfare States in the 21st Century.* Cheltenham: Edward Elgar Publishing.

Greer, S. L. (2004). *Territorial Politics and Health Policy: UK Health Policy in Comparative Perspective.* Manchester: Manchester University Press.

Greer, S. L. (2016). Devolution and Health in the UK: Policy and its Lessons Since 1998. *British Medical Bulletin*, 118(1), 16–24. Retrieved from https://doi.org/10.1093/bmb/ldw013

Greer, S. L., Stewart, E., Ercia, A. and Donnelly, P. (2021). Changing Health Care With, For, Or Against the Public: An Empirical Investigation into the Place of the Public in Health Service Reconfiguration. *Journal of Health Services Research & Policy*, 26(1), 12–19. Retrieved from https://doi.org/10.1177/1355819620935148

Handy, F., Mook, L. and Quarter, J. (2008). The Interchangeability of Paid Staff and Volunteers in Nonprofit Organizations. *Nonprofit and Voluntary Sector Quarterly*, 37(1), 76–92. Retrieved from https://doi.org/10.1177/0899764007303528

Handy, F. and Srinivasan, N. (2004). Valuing Volunteers: An Economic Evaluation of the Net Benefits of Hospital Volunteers. *Nonprofit and Voluntary Sector Quarterly*, 33(1), 28–54. Retrieved from https://doi.org/10.1177/0899764003260961

Hanrahan, P. (2018, September 18). A Modern Volunteering Mission for the NHS. Retrieved from https://www.england.nhs.uk/blog/a-modern-volunteering-mission-for-the-nhs/

Hansen, P. (2022). Decolonization and the Spectre of the Nation-state. *The British Journal of Sociology*, 73(1), 35–49. Retrieved from https://doi.org/10.1111/1468-4446.12909

Harding, S. G. (2004). *The Feminist Standpoint Theory Reader: Intellectual and Political Controversies.* New York: Routledge.

Harris, B. (2004). *The Origins of the British Welfare State: Society, State and Social Welfare in England and Wales, 1800–1945*. London: Bloomsbury Publishing Plc. Retrieved from http://ebookcentral.proquest.com/lib/strath/detail.action?docID=6418711

Harris, B. and Mohan, J. (2021, February). After the Death of Captain Sir Tom Moore, What Role Should Charity Play in Funding the NHS? Retrieved from http://theconversation.com/after-the-death-of-captain-sir-tom-moore-what-role-should-charity-play-in-funding-the-nhs-154693

Harrison, S. and Ahmad, W. (2000). Medical Autonomy and the UK State 1975 to 2025. *Sociology*, 34(1), 129–146.

Haug, J. C. and Gaskins, J. N. (2012). Recruiting and Retaining Volunteer EMTs: From Motivation to Practical Solutions. *International Journal of Sociology and Social Policy*, 32(3/4), 197–213. Retrieved from https://doi.org/10.1108/01443331211214767

Healthcare Improvement Scotland. (2022, October). Data on Volunteer Numbers in NHS Scotland. Unpublished data via personal communication.

Healthwatch. (2019, June). What Does NHS Data About Complaints Tell Us? Retrieved from https://www.healthwatch.co.uk/blog/2019-06-19/what-does-nhs-data-about-complaints-tell-us

Helderman, J.-K. (2015). Making Sense of Complexity: The Contribution of Rudolf Klein to Our Understanding of The New Politics of the NHS. *Health Economics, Policy and Law*, 10(2), 229–235. Retrieved from https://doi.org/10.1017/S1744133114000280

Hellowell, M. and Pollock, A. M. (2009). The Private Financing of NHS Hospitals: Politics, Policy and Practice. *Economic Affairs*, 29(1), 13–19. Retrieved from https://doi.org/10.1111/j.1468-0270.2009.01861.x

Helpforce and UNISON. (2019). *Charter to Strengthen Relations between the Helpforce Programme and Staff in the National Health Service (England)* (No. CU/April 2019/25525/UNP). London: UNISON. Retrieved from https://www.unison.org.uk/content/uploads/2019/04/25525_Joint_unions_health_charter.pdf

Henderson, A. and Jones, R. W. (2021). *Englishness: The Political Force Transforming Britain*. Oxford: Oxford University Press.

Higashi, R. T., Tillack, A., Steinman, M. A., Johnston, C. B. and Harper, G. M. (2013). The 'Worthy' Patient: Rethinking the 'Hidden Curriculum' in Medical Education. *Anthropology & Medicine*, 20(1), 13–23. Retrieved from https://doi.org/10.1080/13648470.2012.747595

Hillman, A. (2014). 'Why Must I Wait?' The Performance of Legitimacy in a Hospital Emergency Department. *Sociology of Health & Illness*, 36(4), 485–499. Retrieved from https://doi.org/10.1111/1467-9566.12072

Hills, J. (2017). *Good Times, Bad Times: The Welfare Myth of Them and Us*. Bristol: Policy Press.

Hitchen, E. and Raynor, R. (2020). Encountering Austerity in Everyday Life: Intensities, Localities, Materialities. *Geoforum*, 110, 186–190. Retrieved from https://doi.org/10.1016/j.geoforum.2019.07.017

Hlavach, L. and Freivogel, W. H. (2011). Ethical Implications of Anonymous Comments Posted to Online News Stories. *Journal of Mass Media Ethics*, 26(1), 21–37. Retrieved from https://doi.org/10.1080/08900523.2011.525190

Hodgkin, P. (2013, 13 December). Five minutes with … the Founder of Patient Opinion. *The Guardian*. Retrieved from https://www.theguardian.com/healthcare-network/2013/dec/13/paul-hodgkin-founder-patient-opinion

Hogg, E. and Smith, A. (2021). *Kickstarting a New Volunteer Revolution*. Cardiff: Royal Voluntary Service. Retrieved from https://www.royalvoluntaryservice.org.uk/media/yvhhp0zl/social_mobility_unleashing_the_power_of_volunteering.pdf

Holmes, H. and Hall, S. M. (2020). *Mundane Methods: Innovative Ways to Research the Everyday*. Manchester: Manchester University Press.

Hook, M. and Mapp, J. (2005). Physician Fundraising: Evolution, Not Revolution. In W. C. McGinly, K. Renzetti, C. Williams and L. Wagner (Eds), *Expanding the Role of Philanthropy in Health Care*. Hoboken, NJ: Jossey-Bass.

Hughes, D. and Griffiths, L. (1997). 'Ruling In' And 'Ruling Out': Two Approaches to the Micro-rationing of Health Care. *Social Science & Medicine*, 44(5), 589–599. Retrieved from https://doi.org/10.1016/S0277-9536(96)00207-9

Hunt, J. (2016). *Welfare Work in Hospitals 1938–2013* (Royal Voluntary Service Heritage Collection) (p 31). Cardiff: Royal Voluntary Service.

Hunter, S. (2016). The Role of Multicultural Fantasies in the Enactment of the State: The English NHS as an Affective Formation. In E. Jupp, J. Pykett and F. M. Smith (Eds), *Emotional States: Sites and Spaces of Affective Governance*. Oxford: Taylor & Francis.

Hutchings, R. (2020). *The Impact of Covid-19 on the Use of Digital Technology in the NHS* (Briefing). London: Nuffield Trust. Retrieved from https://www.actasanitaria.com/uploads/s1/15/56/06/9/the-impact-of-covid-19-on-the-use-of-digital-technology-in-the-nhs-web-2.pdf

Iacobucci, G. (2019). NHS is to Test Scrapping the Four Hour A&E Target. *BMJ*, 364, l1148. Retrieved from https://doi.org/10.1136/bmj.l1148

Igra, M., Kenworthy, N., Luchsinger, C. and Jung, J.-K. (2021). Crowdfunding as a Response to COVID-19: Increasing Inequities at a Time of Crisis. *Social Science & Medicine*, 282, 114105.

International Labour Organization. (2021). *Manual on the Measurement of Volunteer Work*. Geneva: International Labour Organization. Retrieved from https://www.ilo.org/wcmsp5/groups/public/---dgreports/---stat/documents/meetingdocument/wcms_100574.pdf

Ipsos MORI for the King's Fund. (2017). *What Do the Public Think About the NHS?* London: Ipsos MORI. Retrieved from https://www.ipsos.com/sites/default/files/ct/news/documents/2017-09/17-054742-01%20-%20King%27s%20Fund%20NHS%20Expo%20polling%20-%20v1%20-%20INTERNAL%20USE%20ONLY.pdf

Ipsos MORI Public Affairs. (2019). General Election 2019 Polling for the Health Foundation: Public Perceptions of Health and Social Care. London: Ipsos MORI. Retrieved from https://www.health.org.uk/sites/default/files/upload/publications/2019/THF-Public-perceptions-of-health-and-social-care-Dec19.pdf

Isin, E. F. (2009). Citizenship in Flux: The Figure of the Activist Citizen. *Subjectivity: International Journal of Critical Psychology*, 29(1), 367–388. Retrieved from https://doi.org/10.1057/sub.2009.25

Issa, R. and Butt, A. (2022, October 27). NHS Workers Are Striking to Save Lives. Retrieved from https://novaramedia.com/2022/10/27/nhs-workers-are-striking-to-save-lives/

Jagsi, R. (2019). Ethical Issues Involved in Grateful Patient Fundraising. *JAMA*, 321(4), 407–408. Retrieved from https://doi.org/10.1001/jama.2018.18656

Jagsi, R., Griffith, K. A., Carrese, J. A., Collins, M., Kao, A. C., Konrath, S. et al (2020). Public Attitudes Regarding Hospitals and Physicians Encouraging Donations from Grateful Patients. *JAMA*, 324(3), 270–278. Retrieved from https://doi.org/10.1001/jama.2020.9442

Jennings, W. and Wlezien, C. (2018). Election Polling Errors Across Time and Space. *Nature Human Behaviour*, 2(4), 276–283. Retrieved from https://doi.org/10.1038/s41562-018-0315-6

Jensen, C. (2008). Worlds of Welfare Services and Transfers. *Journal of European Social Policy*, 18(2), 151–162. Retrieved from https://doi.org/10.1177/0958928707087591

Jensen, T. (2014). Welfare Commonsense, Poverty Porn and Doxosophy. *Sociological Research Online*, 19(3), 277–283. Retrieved from https://doi.org/10.5153/sro.3441

Jerrim, J. and de Vries, R. (2017). The Limitations of Quantitative Social Science for Informing Public Policy. *Evidence & Policy*, 13(1), 117–133. Retrieved from https://doi.org/10.1332/174426415X14431000856662

Jezierska, K. and Sörbom, A. (2021). Proximity and Distance: Think Tanks Handling the Independence Paradox. *Governance*, 34(2), 395–411. Retrieved from https://doi.org/10.1111/gove.12503

Jones, L. (2015). What Does a Hospital Mean? *Journal of Health Services Research & Policy*, 20(4), 254–256.

Jones, L., Fraser, A. and Stewart, E. (2019). Exploring the Neglected and Hidden Dimensions of Large-scale Healthcare Change. *Sociology of Health & Illness*, 41(7), 1221–1235. Retrieved from https://doi.org/10.1111/1467-9566.12923

Jordan, J. (2013). Policy Feedback and Support for the Welfare State. *Journal of European Social Policy*, 23(2), 134–148. Retrieved from https://doi.org/10.1177/0958928712471224

Jupp, E. (2022). *Care, Crisis and Activism: The Politics of Everyday Life*. Bristol: Policy Press.

Kamerāde, D. and Paine, A. E. (2014). Volunteering and Employability: Implications for Policy and Practice. *Voluntary Sector Review*, 5(2), 259–273. Retrieved from https://doi.org/10.1332/204080514X14013593888736

Kar, P. (2020). Partha Kar: To Tackle Racism, the NHS Needs Policies with Teeth. *BMJ*, 369, m2583. Retrieved from https://doi.org/10.1136/bmj.m2583

Katikireddi, S. V., Higgins, M., Smith, K. E. and Williams, G. (2013). Health Inequalities: The Need to Move Beyond Bad Behaviours. *Journal of Epidemiology and Community Health*, 67(9), 715–716. Retrieved from https://doi.org/10.1136/jech-2012-202064

Kenworthy, N. (2021). Like a Grinding Stone: How Crowdfunding Platforms Create, Perpetuate, and Value Health Inequities. *Medical Anthropology Quarterly*, 35(3). Retrieved from https://doi.org/10.1111/maq.12639

Kenworthy, N., Jung, J.-K. and Hops, E. (2022). Struggling, Helping and Adapting: Crowdfunding Motivations and Outcomes During the Early US COVID-19 Pandemic. Sociology of Health & Illness, 45(2), 298–316. Retrieved from https://doi.org/10.1111/1467-9566.13568

Kerr, A., Chekar, C. K., Ross, E., Swallow, J. and Cunningham-Burley, S. (2021). *Personalised Cancer Medicine: Future Crafting in the Genomic Era*. Manchester: Manchester University Press.

Kerr, A., Chekar, C. K., Swallow, J., Ross, E. and Cunningham-Burley, S. (2021). Accessing Targeted Therapies for Cancer: Self and Collective Advocacy Alongside and Beyond Mainstream Cancer Charities. *New Genetics and Society*, 40(1), 112–131. Retrieved from https://doi.org/10.1080/14636778.2020.1868986

Kerr, A., Cunningham-Burley, S. and Tutton, R. (2007). Shifting Subject Positions Experts and Lay People in Public Dialogue. *Social Studies of Science*, 37(3), 385–411. Retrieved from https://doi.org/10.1177/0306312706068492

Ketola, M. and Nordensvard, J. (2018). Reviewing the Relationship Between Social Policy and the Contemporary Populist Radical Right: Welfare Chauvinism, Welfare Nation State and Social Citizenship. *Journal of International and Comparative Social Policy*, 34(3), 172–187. Retrieved from https://doi.org/10.1080/21699763.2018.1521863

Kielmann, K., Hutchinson, E. and MacGregor, H. (2022). Health Systems Performance or Performing Health Systems? Anthropological Engagement with Health Systems Research. *Social Science & Medicine*, 300. Retrieved from https://doi.org/10.1016/j.socscimed.2022.114838

King Edward's Hospital Fund for London. (1977). *Evidence to the Royal Commission on the National Health Service*. London: King Edward's Hospital Fund for London. Retrieved from https://archive.kingsfund.org.uk/conc ern/published_works/000003196?locale=en#?cv=30&xywh=-2451,-114,6203,2025&p=0

King's Fund. (2017). What Does the Public Think About the NHS? Retrieved from https://www.kingsfund.org.uk/publications/what-does-public-think-about-nhs

King's Fund. (2022). The NHS Budget and How it Has Changed. Retrieved from https://www.kingsfund.org.uk/projects/nhs-in-a-nutshell/nhs-budget

Klein, R. (2010). *The New Politics of the NHS: From Creation to Reinvention* (6th ed.). Oxford: Radcliffe.

Klein, R. (2013). *The New Politics of the NHS, Seventh Edition* (7th edn). London: CRC Press.

Klein, R. and Rafferty, A.-M. (2004). Rorschach Politics: Tony Blair and the Third Way. In N. Deakin, C. J. Finer and B. Matthews (Eds), *Welfare and the State: Welfare Futures*. Oxford: Taylor & Francis.

Knox, A. (2017). Public Perspectives on the NHS. Retrieved from https://www.nuffieldtrust.org.uk/news-item/public-perspectives-on-the-nhs

Kyriakides, C. and Virdee, S. (2003). Migrant Labour, Racism and the British National Health Service. *Ethnicity & Health*, 8(4), 283–305. Retrieved from https://doi.org/10.1080/13557850310001631731

Labov, W. (1997). Some Further Steps in Narrative Analysis. *Journal of Narrative and Life History*, 7(1–4), 395–415. Retrieved from https://doi.org/10.1075/jnlh.7.49som

Langstrup, H. (2013). Chronic Care Infrastructures and the Home. *Sociology of Health & Illness*, 35(7), 1008–1022. Retrieved from https://doi.org/10.1111/1467-9566.12013

Larsen, E. G. (2020). Personal Politics? Healthcare Policies, Personal Experiences and Government Attitudes. *Journal of European Social Policy*, 30(4), 467–479. Retrieved from https://doi.org/10.1177/0958928720904319

Latour, B. (2005). From Realpolitik to Dingpolitik or How to Make Things Public. In B. Latour and P. Weibel (Eds), *Making Things Public: Atmospheres of Democracy*. Cambridge, MA: MIT Press.

Lattimer, M. (1996). *The Gift of Health: The NHS, Charity and the Mixed Economy of Healthcare*. London: Directory of Social Change.

Law, J. (2009). Seeing Like a Survey. *Cultural Sociology*, 3(2), 239–256. Retrieved from https://doi.org/10.1177/1749975509105533

Leduc-Cummings, I., Starrs, C. J. and Perry, J. C. (2020). Idealization. In V. Zeigler-Hill and T. K. Shackelford (Eds), *Encyclopedia of Personality and Individual Differences* (pp 2129–2132). Cham: Springer International Publishing.

Leitch, J. (2019, August 15). Leadership of Volunteering in NHS Scotland: Recommendations. Retrieved from https://www.hisengage.scot/media/1599/leadership-of-volunteering-letter-from-jason-leitch-15-august-2019.pdf

Lent, A., Pollard, G. and Studdert, J. (2022, 12 July). A Community-Powered NHS. Retrieved from https://www.newlocal.org.uk/publications/community-powered-nhs/

Lewis, G., Gewirtz, S. and Clarke, J. (2000). *Rethinking Social Policy*. London: SAGE.

Lindsey, R., Mohan, J., Bulloch, S. and Metcalfe, E. (2018). *Continuity and Change in Voluntary Action: Patterns, Trends and Understandings*. Bristol: Policy Press.

Lintern, S. and Wheeler, C. (2022, 29 August). Britain Falls Out of love with the NHS: Poll Reveals Three in Five Now Expect Delays. *The Times*. Retrieved from https://www.thetimes.co.uk/article/britain-falls-out-of-love-with-the-nhs-poll-reveals-three-in-five-now-expect-delays-v8mnz0tx3

Llanwarne, N., Newbould, J., Burt, J., Campbell, J. L. and Roland, M. (2017). Wasting the Doctor's Time? A Video-elicitation Interview Study with Patients in Primary Care. *Social Science & Medicine*, 176, 113–122. Retrieved from https://doi.org/10.1016/j.socscimed.2017.01.025

Locock, L., Skea, Z., Alexander, G., Hiscox, C., Laidlaw, L. and Shepherd, J. (2020). Anonymity, Veracity and Power in Online Patient Feedback: A Quantitative and Qualitative Analysis of Staff Responses to Patient Comments on the 'Care Opinion' Platform in Scotland. *Digital Health*, 6. Retrieved from https://doi.org/10.1177/2055207619899520

Lorne, C. (2022). Repoliticising National Policy Mobilities: Resisting the Americanization of Universal Healthcare. *Environment and Planning C: Politics and Space*, Online First. Retrieved from https://doi.org/10.1177/23996544211068724

Lowe, R. (1990). The Second World War, Consensus, and the Foundation of the Welfare State. *Twentieth Century British History*, 1(2), 152–182. Retrieved from https://doi.org/10.1093/tcbh/1.2.152

Lucius-Hoene, G., Holmberg, C. and Meyer, T. (2018). *Illness Narratives in Practice: Potentials and Challenges of Using Narratives in Health-Related Contexts*. Oxford: Oxford University Press.

Lupton, D. (2014). The Commodification of Patient Opinion: The Digital Patient Experience Economy in the Age of Big Data. *Sociology of Health & Illness*, 36(6), 856–869.

Madden, H., Harris, J., Blickem, C., Harrison, R. and Timpson, H. (2017). 'Always Paracetamol, They Give Them Paracetamol for everything': A Qualitative Study Examining Eastern European Migrants' Experiences of the UK Health Service. *BMC Health Services Research*, 17(1), 604. Retrieved from https://doi.org/10.1186/s12913-017-2526-3

Madden, M. and Speed, E. (2017). Beware Zombies and Unicorns: Toward Critical Patient and Public Involvement in Health Research in a Neoliberal Context. *Frontiers in Sociology*, 2. Retrieved from https://doi.org/10.3389/fsoc.2017.00007

Mahase, E. (2021). Covid-19: NHS Test and Trace Failed Despite 'Eye Watering' Budget, MPs Conclude. *BMJ*, 375, n2606. Retrieved from https://doi.org/10.1136/bmj.n2606

Mak, K. A., Sheikh, A.-R., Grieve, S. and Mendonca, C. (2021). Lessons Learnt from Medical Students' Experiences of Volunteering in the NHS During the COVID-19 Pandemic. *Future Healthcare Journal*, 8(3), e734–e734.

Malby, R., Boyle, D. and Crilly, T. (2017). *Can Volunteering Help Create Better Health and Care. An Evidence Review*. London: London South Bank University. Retrieved from https://doi.org/10.18744/PUB.001625

Maller, C. J. (2015). Understanding Health Through Social Practices: Performance and Materiality in Everyday Life. *Sociology of Health & Illness*, 37(1), 52–66. Retrieved from https://doi.org/10.1111/1467-9566.12178

Mao, G., Fernandes-Jesus, M., Ntontis, E. and Drury, J. (2021). What Have We Learned About COVID-19 Volunteering in the UK? A Rapid Review of the Literature. *BMC Public Health*, 21(1), 1470. Retrieved from https://doi.org/10.1186/s12889-021-11390-8

Marmor, T. (2008). Review of 'The New Politics of the NHS: From Creation to Reinvention'. *Journal of Health Politics, Policy and Law*, 33(2), 329–332. Retrieved from https://doi.org/10.1215/03616878-2007-057

Marmor, T. R., Okma, K. G. H. and Latham, S. R. (2010) National Values, Institutions and Health Policies: What do they Imply for Medicare Reform?, *Journal of Comparative Policy Analysis: Research and Practice*, 12(1–2), 179–196. DOI: 10.1080/13876980903076286

Marmot, M. (2010). *Fair Society, Healthy Lives: Strategic Review of Health Inequalities in England post-2010* (The Marmot Review). London: The Marmot Review. Retrieved from http://www.instituteofhealthequity.org/projects/fair-society-healthy-lives-the-marmot-review

Martin, D., Nettleton, S., Buse, C., Prior, L. and Twigg, J. (2015). Architecture and Health Care: A Place for Sociology. *Sociology of Health & Illness*, 37(7), 1007–1022. Retrieved from https://doi.org/10.1111/1467-9566.12284

Martin, G. P., Chew, S. and Dixon-Woods, M. (2021). Why Do Systems for Responding to Concerns and Complaints So Often Fail Patients, Families and healthcare staff? A Qualitative Study. *Social Science & Medicine*, 287, 114375. Retrieved from https://doi.org/10.1016/j.socscimed.2021.114375

Mason, J. (2017). *Qualitative Researching* (3rd edn). Thousand Oaks, CA: SAGE Publications Ltd.

Mason, R. (2022, 19 August). Revealed: Liz Truss Personally Supported Cuts to NHS and Doctors' Pay. *The Guardian*. Retrieved from https://www.theguardian.com/politics/2022/aug/19/revealed-liz-truss-supported-cuts-to-nhs-and-doctors-pay-in-thinktank-report

Matthews, K. and Nazroo, J. (2021). The Impact of Volunteering and Its Characteristics on Well-being After State Pension Age: Longitudinal Evidence From the English Longitudinal Study of Ageing. *The Journals of Gerontology: Series B*, 76(3), 632–641. Retrieved from https://doi.org/10.1093/geronb/gbaa146

Maybin, J. (2016). *Producing Health Policy Knowledge and Knowing in Government Policy Work*. London: Palgrave Macmillan UK.

Mays, N. and Pope, C. (2000). Qualitative Research in Health Care: Assessing Quality in Qualitative Research. *BMJ*, 320(7226), 50–52.

Mazanderani, F., Kirkpatrick, S. F., Ziebland, S., Locock, L. and Powell, J. (2021). Caring for Care: Online Feedback in the Context of Public Healthcare Services. *Social Science & Medicine*, 285, 114280. Retrieved from https://doi.org/10.1016/j.socscimed.2021.114280

Mazanderani, F. and Powell, J. F. (2013). Using the Internet as a Resource for Exploring Patients' Experiences. In S. Ziebland, A. Coulter, J. Calabrese and L. Locock (Eds), *Understanding and Using Health Experiences: Improving Patient Care*. Oxford: Oxford University Press (pp 94–103). Retrieved from https://doi.org/10.1093/acprof:oso/9780199665372.003.0010

McCartney, M. (2016). *The State of Medicine: Keeping the Promise of the NHS* (1st edn). Pinter & Martin.

McCartney, M. (2022). The Modern Medical Memoir. *The Lancet*, 399(10328), 901. Retrieved from https://doi.org/10.1016/S0140-6736(22)00386-5

McGinly, W. C. (2008). The Maturing Role of Philanthropy in Healthcare. *Frontiers of Health Services Management; Chicago*, 24(4), 11–22.

McHale, J., Speakman, E. M., Hervey, T. and Flear, M. (2021). Health Law and Policy, Devolution and Brexit. *Regional Studies*, 55(9), 1561–1570. Retrieved from https://doi.org/10.1080/00343404.2020.1736538

McKee, H. A. and Porter, J. E. (2009). *The Ethics of Internet Research: A Rhetorical, Case-based Process*. Lausanne: Peter Lang.

Mcmurray, M. (2008). *The Formation and Founding of the Women's Voluntary Services for A.R.P.* (Royal Voluntary Service Heritage Collection) (p 12). Retrieved from Cardiff: Royal Voluntary Service:

Meer, N. (2015). Looking Up in Scotland? Multinationalism, Multiculturalism and Political Elites. *Ethnic and Racial Studies*, 38(9), 1477–1496. Retrieved from https://doi.org/10.1080/01419870.2015.1005642

Meer, N. (2022). Who Still Needs the Nation? Empire, Identity and the British Welfare State. *The British Journal of Sociology*, 73(1). Retrieved from https://doi.org/10.1111/1468-4446.12910

Merrison, A. (1979). *Royal Commission on the NHS*. Retrieved from https://www.sochealth.co.uk/national-health-service/royal-commission-on-the-national-health-service-contents/royal-commission-on-the-nhs-chapter-11/

Merry, S. E. (2016). *The Seductions of Quantification: Measuring Human Rights, Gender Violence, and Sex Trafficking*. Chicago, IL: University of Chicago Press.

Millar, J. (2022). 'Relations of Extraction': Some Issues for Social Policy. *British Journal of Sociology*, 73(1), 60–66.

Miller, O. (2020). More Resource Will Be Required to Support NHS Volunteers. Retrieved from https://www.kent.ac.uk/news/society/24829/expert-comment-more-resource-will-be-required-to-support-nhs-volunteers

Millward, G. (2023). 'Its Many Workers and Subscribers Feel That Their Services Can Still Be of Benefit': Hospital Leagues of Friends in the English West Midlands, c. 1948–1998. *Social History of Medicine*, Advance Article.

Mohammed, S., Peter, E., Killackey, T. and Maciver, J. (2021). The 'Nurse as Hero' Discourse in the COVID-19 Pandemic: A Poststructural Discourse Analysis. *International Journal of Nursing Studies*, 117, 103887.

Mohan, J. (2002). *Planning, Markets and Hospitals*. Abingdon: Routledge.

Mohan, J. and Gorsky, M. (2001). *Don't Look Back? Voluntary and Charitable Finance of Hospitals*. London: Office of Health Economics.

Möller, C. and Abnett, H. (under review). Strategic Distinctiveness: Awakening the 'Sleeping Giants' of England and Wales's NHS Charities. *Voluntary Sector Review*.

Montgomery, C. M., Powell, J., Mahtani, K. and Boylan, A.-M. (2022). Turning the Gaze: Digital Patient Feedback and the Silent Pathology of the NHS. *Sociology of Health & Illness*, 44(2), 290–307.

Moran, M. (1999). *Governing the Health Care State: A Comparative Study of the United Kingdom, the United States, and Germany*. Manchester: Manchester University Press.

More Partnership. (2020). Case Study: NHS Charities Together. Retrieved from http://www.morepartnership.com/casestudy-nhsct.html

Mortimore, R. and Wells, A. (2017). The Polls and Their Context. In D. Wring, R. Mortimore and S. Atkinson (Eds), *Political Communication in Britain: Polling, Campaigning and Media in the 2015 General Election* (pp 19–38). Cham: Springer International Publishing. Retrieved from https://doi.org/10.1007/978-3-319-40934-4_3

Munro, J. (2015). The Research Potential of Patient Opinion. Retrieved from https://www.careopinion.org.uk/blogposts/382/the-research-potential-of-patient-opinion

NatCen Social Research. (2022). Funding British Social Attitudes. Retrieved from https://www.bsa.natcen.ac.uk/about/funding.aspx

Naylor, C., Mundle, C., Weaks, L. and Buck, D. (2013). *Volunteering in Health and Care*. London: Kings Fund. Retrieved from http://www.kingsfund.org.uk/publications/volunteering-health-and-care

NCVO. (2020, July). Volunteering Round-up: July 2020. Retrieved from https://blogs.ncvo.org.uk/2020/07/29/volunteering-round-up-july-2020/

Needham, C. (2009). Editorial: Consumerism in Public Services. *Public Money & Management*, 29(2), 79–81. Retrieved from https://doi.org/10.1080/09540960902767923

NESTA. (2013). People Powered Health Programme. Retrieved from https://www.nesta.org.uk/project/people-powered-health/

New Philanthropy Capital. (2019). Learning Together as a Sector: NHS Charities Using Shared Measurement. London: Imperial Health Charity. Retrieved from https://www.nhscharitiestogether.co.uk/wp-content/uploads/2019/09/NPC_sharedmeasurement_report_WEB.pdf

Newbigging, K. (2016). Blowin' in the Wind: The Involvement of People Who Use Services, Carers and the Public in Health and Social Care. In M. Exworthy, R. Mannion and M. Powell (Eds), *Dismantling the NHS? Evaluating the Impact of Health Reforms*. Bristol: Policy Press.

Newman, J. (2012). *Working the Spaces of Power: Activism, Neoliberalism and Gendered Labour*. London: A&C Black.

Newman, J. and Clarke, J. (2009). *Publics, Politics and Power: Remaking the Public in Public Services*. Thousand Oaks, CA: SAGE.

NHS Careers. (2022). NHS Reservists. Retrieved from https://www.healthcareers.nhs.uk/we-are-nhs/nhs-reservists

NHS Charities Together. (2021). Our Covid-19 Appeal. Retrieved from https://nhscharitiestogether.co.uk/our-covid-19-appeal/

NHS Charities Together. (2022a). About NHS Charities Together. Retrieved from https://nhscharitiestogether.co.uk/what-we-do-1/

NHS Charities Together. (2022b). Be There for Them. Retrieved from https://nhscharitiestogether.co.uk/be-there-for-them/

NHS England. (2013). *The NHS Constitution for England*. London: Department of Health. Retrieved from https://assets.publishing.service.gov.uk/gov ernment/uploads/system/uploads/attachment_data/file/170656/NHS_ Constitution.pdf

NHS England. (2022a). About the NHS Birthday. Retrieved from https:// www.england.nhs.uk/nhsbirthday/about-the-nhs-birthday/

NHS England. (2022b). NHS Citizen. Retrieved from https://www.engl and.nhs.uk/get-involved/get-involved/how/nhs-citizen/

NHS England. (2022c). NHS Identity Guidelines. Retrieved from https:// www.england.nhs.uk/nhsidentity/

NHS England. (2022d). Major Drive Launched to Recruit NHS Reservists. Retrieved from https://www.england.nhs.uk/2022/03/major-drive-launc hed-to-recruit-nhs-reservists/

NHS Inform. (2022). Volunteering with the NHS. Retrieved from https:// www.nhsinform.scot/care-support-and-rights/nhs-services/volunteering/ volunteering-with-the-nhs

NHS Race and Health Observatory. (2022). About Us. Retrieved from https://www.nhsrho.org/about-us/

NHS Scotland. (2015). *Realistic Medicine: Chief Medical Officer's Report 2014– 2015*. Edinburgh: The Scottish Government.

NHS Volunteer Responders. (2020). NHS Volunteer Responders. Retrieved from https://nhsvolunteerresponders.org.uk/index.aspx

NHS Wales. (2022). Work, Volunteering and Work Experience Questions. Retrieved from https://www.wales.nhs.uk/ourservices/contactus/ workvolunteeringandworkexperiencequestions

Nuffield Trust. (2018). NHS Estates: Viewpoints. Retrieved from https:// www.nuffieldtrust.org.uk/resource/nhs-estates-viewpoints

Ocloo, J. E. (2010). Harmed Patients Gaining Voice: Challenging Dominant Perspectives in the Construction of Medical Harm and Patient Safety Reforms. *Social Science & Medicine*, 71(3), 510–516.

O'Donohue, W. and Nelson, L. G. (2009). The Psychological Contracts of Australian Hospital Volunteer Workers. *Australian Journal on Volunteering*, 14(9), EJ.

Oliver, D. (2021). David Oliver: Lack of PPE Betrays NHS Clinical Staff. *BMJ*, 372, n438. Retrieved from https://doi.org/10.1136/bmj.n438

Olza, I., Koller, V., Ibarretxe-Antuñano, I., Pérez-Sobrino, P. and Semino, E. (2021). The #ReframeCovid initiative: From Twitter to society via metaphor. *Metaphor and the Social World*. 11(1), 99–121.

Or, Z., Cases, C., Lisac, M., Vrangbæk, K., Winblad, U. and Bevan, G. (2010). Are Health Problems Systemic? Politics of Access and Choice Under Beveridge and Bismarck Systems. *Health Economics, Policy and Law*, 5(3), 269–293. Retrieved from https://doi.org/10.1017/S1744133110000034

Osborne, T. and Rose, N. (1999). Do the Social Sciences Create Phenomena? The Example of Public Opinion Research. *The British Journal of Sociology*, 50(3), 367–396. Retrieved from https://doi.org/10.1111/j.1468-4446.1999.00367.x

Özkazanç-Pan, B. and Pullen, A. (2020). Gendered Labour and Work, Even in Pandemic Times. *Gender, Work & Organization*, 27(5), 675–676. Retrieved from https://doi.org/10.1111/gwao.12516

Paine, A. E., Kamerāde, D., Mohan, J. and Davidson, D. (2019). Communities as 'Renewable Energy' for Healthcare Services? A Multimethods Study into the Form, Scale and Role of Voluntary Support for Community Hospitals in England. *BMJ Open*, 9(10), e030243. Retrieved from https://doi.org/10.1136/bmjopen-2019-030243

Painter, J. (2006). Prosaic Geographies of Stateness. *Political Geography*, 25(7), 752–774. Retrieved from https://doi.org/10.1016/j.polgeo.2006.07.004

Papanicolas, I., Mossialos, E., Gundersen, A., Woskie, L. and Jha, A. K. (2019). Performance of UK National Health Service Compared with Other High Income Countries: Observational Study. *BMJ*, 367, l6326. Retrieved from https://doi.org/10.1136/bmj.l6326

Parsons, T. (1951). *The Social System*. New York: Free Press.

Paton, C. (2022). *NHS Reform and Health Politics in the UK: Revolution, Counter-Revolution and Covid Crisis* (1st edn). Basingstoke: Palgrave Macmillan.

Paulus, T. M. and Roberts, K. R. (2018). Crowdfunding a 'Real-life Superhero': The Construction of Worthy Bodies in Medical Campaign Narratives, *Discourse, Context & Media*, 21, 64–72. Retrieved from https://doi.org/10.1016/j.dcm.2017.09.008

Pearce, R. (2018). *Understanding Trans Health: Discourse, Power and Possibility*. Bristol: Policy Press.

Pickell, Z., Gu, K. and Williams, A. M. (2020). Virtual Volunteers: The Importance of Restructuring Medical Volunteering During the COVID-19 Pandemic. *Medical Humanities*, 46(4), 537–540. Retrieved from https://doi.org/10.1136/medhum-2020-011956

Pickett, K. and Wilkinson, R. (2015). Spirit Level: A Case Study of the Public Dissemination of Health Inequalities Research in K. E. Smith, C. Bambra and S. E. Hill (Eds), *Health Inequalities: Critical Perspectives*. Oxford: Oxford University Press.

Pickles, K. (2019, 1 January). Mail Reader Recruits Sees 2,500 Sign Up to Be NHS Volunteers. *Mail Online*. Retrieved from https://www.dailymail.co.uk/news/article-6543589/Final-surge-Mail-reader-recruits-sees-2-500-sign-NHS-volunteers-just-24-hours.html

Piggott, R. (2022). Hospital Sunday and the New National Health Service: An End to 'The Voluntary Spirit' in England? *Studies in Church History*, 58, 372–393. Retrieved from https://doi.org/10.1017/stc.2022.18

Pitkeathley, J., Volunteer Centre, King's Fund Centre and Gay, P. (1982). *Mobilising Voluntary Resources: The Work of the Voluntary Service Coordinator.* London: King Edward's Hospital Fund for London

Pols, J. (2005). Enacting Appreciations: Beyond the Patient Perspective. *Health Care Analysis*, 13(3), 203–21. Retrieved from http://dx.doi.org/10.1007/s10728-005-6448-6

Powell, M. (2007). *Understanding the Mixed Economy of Welfare.* Bristol: Policy Press.

Powell, M. (2015). Who Killed the English National Health Service? *International Journal of Health Policy and Management*, 4(5), 267–269. Retrieved from https://doi.org/10.15171/ijhpm.2015.72

Prainsack, B. (2020). Solidarity in Times of Pandemics. *Democratic Theory*, 7(2), 124–133. Retrieved from https://doi.org/10.3167/dt.2020.070215

Prainsack, B. and Buyx, A. (2017). *Solidarity in Biomedicine and Beyond.* Cambridge: Cambridge University Press.

Prochaska, F. (1997). *Philanthropy and the Hospitals of London: The King's Fund, 1897–1990* (1st edn). Oxford: Oxford University Press.

Pushkar, P. and Tomkow, L. (2021). Clinician-led Evidence-based Activism: A Critical Analysis. *Critical Public Health*, 31(2), 235–244. Retrieved from https://doi.org/10.1080/09581596.2020.1841112

Rabeharisoa, V., Moreira, T. and Akrich, M. (2014). Evidence-based Activism: Patients', Users' and Activists' Groups in Knowledge Society. *BioSocieties*, 9(2), 111–128. Retrieved from https://doi.org/10.1057/biosoc.2014.2

Ramsden, S. and Cresswell, R. (2019). First Aid and Voluntarism in England, 1945–85. *Twentieth Century British History*, 30(4), 504–530. Retrieved from https://doi.org/10.1093/tcbh/hwy043

Reader, T. W., Gillespie, A. and Roberts, J. (2014). Patient Complaints in Healthcare Systems: A Systematic Review and Coding Taxonomy. *BMJ Quality & Safety*, 23(8), 678–689. Retrieved from https://doi.org/10.1136/bmjqs-2013-002437

Reed, S., Oung, C., Davies, J., Dayan, M. and Scobie, S. (2021). *Integrating Health and Social Care* (Research report). London: Nuffield Trust.

Reibling, N., Ariaans, M. and Wendt, C. (2019). Worlds of Healthcare: A Healthcare System Typology of OECD Countries. *Health Policy*, 123(7), 611–620. Retrieved from https://doi.org/10.1016/j.healthpol.2019.05.001

Research Works Limited. (2016). *NHS Identity Research: Phase One and Two Combined Research Report.* Leeds: NHS England. Retrieved from https://www.england.nhs.uk/nhsidentity/wp-content/uploads/sites/38/2016/08/NHS-Identity-Research-phase-one-and-two.pdf

Riessman, C. K. (2008). *Narrative Methods for the Human Sciences*. London: SAGE.

Robert, G., Cornwell, J. and Black, N. (2018). Friends and Family Test Should No Longer Be Mandatory. *BMJ*, 360, k367. Retrieved from https://doi.org/10.1136/bmj.k367

Rochester, C. (2013). *Rediscovering Voluntary Action: The Beat of a Different Drum*. Basingstoke: Palgrave Macmillan UK. Retrieved from https://link.springer.com/book/10.1057/9781137029461

Rochester, C., Paine, A. E., Howlett, S. and Zimmeck, M. (2010). Defending the Spirit of Volunteering from Formalisation. In C. Rochester, A. E. Paine, S. Howlett and M. Zimmeck (Eds), *Volunteering and Society in the 21st Century* (pp 220–232). London: Palgrave Macmillan UK. Retrieved from https://doi.org/10.1057/9780230279438_16

Rogers, K. B. and Robinson, D. T. (2014). Measuring Affect and Emotions. *Handbook of the Sociology of Emotions: Volume II*, 283–303. Retrieved from https://doi.org/10.1007/978-94-017-9130-4_14

Rosen, M. (2020). Foreword. In D. Alma and K. Amiel (Eds), *These Are The Hands: Poems from the Heart of the NHS*. Oswestry: Fair Acre Press.

Rosen, M. (2021). *Many Different Kinds of Love: A Story of Life, Death and the NHS*. London: Random House.

Ross, S., Fenney, D., Ward, D. and Buck, D. (2018). *The Role of Volunteers in the NHS: Views from the Front Line*. London: King's Fund. Retrieved from https://www.kingsfund.org.uk/sites/default/files/2018-12/Role_volunteers_NHS_December_2018.pdf

Rossner, M. and Meher, M. (2014). Emotions in Ritual Theories. In J. E. Stets and J. H. Turner (Eds), *Handbook of the Sociology of Emotions: Volume II* (pp 283–303). Dordrecht: Springer. Retrieved from https://link.springer.com/chapter/10.1007/978-94-017-9130-4_14

Rowland, P., McMillan, S., McGillicuddy, P. and Richards, J. (2017). What is 'the Patient Perspective' in Patient Engagement Programs? Implicit Logics and Parallels to Feminist Theories. *Health*, 21(1), 76–92. Retrieved from https://doi.org/10.1177/1363459316644494

Ruane, S. (1997). Public–private Boundaries and the Transformation of the NHS. *Critical Social Policy*, 17(51), 53–78.

Sanghera, S. (2021). *Empireland: How Imperialism Has Shaped Modern Britain* (1st edn). London: Viking.

Saunders, J. (2022). The Making of 'NHS staff' as a Worker Identity 1948–85. In J. Crane and J. Hand (Eds), Posters, Protests, and Prescriptions: Cultural Histories of the National Health Service in Britain. Manchester: Manchester University Press.

Schneider, S. M., Roots, Ave and Rathmann, Katharina. (2021). Health Outcomes and Health Inequalities. In E. M. Immergut, K. M. Anderson, C. Devitt and T. Popic (Eds), *Health Politics in Europe*. Oxford: Oxford University Press. Retrieved from https://doi.org/10.1093/oso/978019 8860525.003.0001

Schneider, W. H., Meslin, E. M. and Daniken, C. (2008). Health and Philanthropy: Leveraging Change. *Nonprofit and Voluntary Sector Quarterly*, 37(1_suppl), 3S–5S. Retrieved from https://doi.org/10.1177/089976400 7310540

Seaton, A. (2015). Against the 'Sacred Cow': NHS Opposition and the Fellowship for Freedom in Medicine, 1948–72. *Twentieth Century British History*, 26(3), 424–449. Retrieved from https://doi.org/10.1093/tcbh/hwv011

Semino, E. (2021). 'Not Soldiers but Fire-fighters' – Metaphors and COVID-19. *Health Communication*, 36(1), 50–58. Retrieved from https://doi.org/10.1080/10410236.2020.1844989

Shapiro, J. (2011). Illness Narratives: Reliability, Authenticity and the Empathic Witness. *Medical Humanities*, 37(2), 68–72. Retrieved from https://doi.org/10.1136/jmh.2011.007328

Shaw, S. E., Russell, J., Greenhalgh, T. and Korica, M. (2014). Thinking About Think Tanks in Health Care: A Call for a New Research Agenda. *Sociology of Health & Illness*, 36(3), 447–461. Retrieved from https://doi.org/10.1111/1467-9566.12071

Shaw, S. E., Russell, J., Parsons, W. and Greenhalgh, T. (2015). The View from Nowhere? How Think Tanks Work to Shape Health Policy. *Critical Policy Studies*, 9(1), 58–77. Retrieved from https://doi.org/10.1080/19460 171.2014.964278

Sheard, S. (2011). A Creature of its Time: The Critical History of the Creation of the British NHS. *Michael Quarterly*, 8, 428–441.

Sheard, S. (2022). 'I'm afraid, there's no NHS'. In J. Crane and J. Hand (Eds), *Posters, Protests, and Prescriptions: Cultural Histories of the National Health Service in Britain: 34*. Manchester: Manchester University Press.

Smith, J., Walshe, K. and Hunter, D. J. (2001). The 'Redisorganisation' of the NHS: Another Reorganisation Involving Unhappy Managers Can Only Worsen the Service. *BMJ*, 323(7324), 1262–1263. Retrieved from https://doi.org/10.1136/bmj.323.7324.1262

Smith, K. and Hellowell, M. (2012). Beyond Rhetorical Differences: A Cohesive Account of Post-devolution Developments in UK Health Policy. *Social Policy & Administration*, 46(2), 178–198.

Social Care Future. (2022). What is #SocialCareFuture. Retrieved from https://socialcarefuture.org.uk/

South, J., White, J. and Gamsu, M. (2012). *People-Centred Public Health*. Bristol: Policy Press.

Speed, E., Crawford, L. and Rutherford, A. (2022). Voluntary Action and the Pandemic Across the UK. In I. Hardill, J. Grotz and L. Crawford (Eds), *Mobilising Voluntary Action in the UK: Learning from the Pandemic* (pp 19–39). Bristol: Policy Press.

Speed, E., Davison, C. and Gunnell, C. (2016). The Anonymity Paradox in Patient Engagement: Reputation, Risk and Web-based Public Feedback. *Medical Humanities*, 42(2), 135–140. Retrieved from https://doi.org/10.1136/medhum-2015-010823

Speed, E. and Mannion, R. (2020). Populism and Health Policy: Three International Case Studies of Right-wing Populist Policy Frames. *Sociology of Health & Illness*, 42(8), 1967–1981. Retrieved from https://doi.org/10.1111/1467-9566.13173

St John Ambulance. (2021). NHS Cadets Homepage. Retrieved from https://www.sja.org.uk/get-involved/young-people/nhs-cadets/

Stanley, L. (2022). *Britain Alone: How a Decade of Conflict Remade the Nation.* Manchester: Manchester University Press.

Stewart, E. (2016). *Publics and Their Health Systems: Rethinking Participation.* Basingstoke: Palgrave Macmillan.

Stewart, E. (2019). A Sociology of Public Responses to Hospital Change and Closure. *Sociology of Health & Illness*, 41(7), 1251–1269. Retrieved from https://doi.org/10.1111/1467-9566.12896

Stewart, E. (2021). Fugitive Coproduction: Conceptualising Informal Community Practices in Scotland's Hospitals. *Social Policy & Administration*, 55(7). Retrieved from https://doi.org/10.1111/spol.12727

Stewart, E. A. (2012). *Governance, Participation and Avoidance: Everyday Public Involvement in the Scottish NHS* (PhD thesis). Edinburgh: University of Edinburgh.

Stewart, E. and Dodworth, K. (2020). Public Fundraising for the NHS, and its Discomforts. Retrieved from https://www.cost-ofliving.net/public-fundraising-for-the-nhs-and-its-discomforts/

Stewart, E., Dodworth, K. and Ercia, A. (2022). The Everyday Work of Hospital Campaigns: Public Knowledge and Activism in the UK's National Health Services. In J. Crane and J. Hand (Eds), *Posters, Protests, and Prescriptions: Cultural Histories of the National Health Service in Britain.* Manchester: Manchester University Press.

Stewart, E., Greer, S. L., Ercia, A. and Donnelly, P. D. (2020). Transforming Health Care: The Policy and Politics of Service Reconfiguration in the UK's Four Health Systems. *Health Economics, Policy and Law*, 15(3), 289–307. Retrieved from https://doi.org/10.1017/S1744133119000148

Stewart, E., Nonhebel, A., Möller, C. and Bassett, K. (2022). Doing 'Our Bit': Solidarity, Inequality, and COVID-19 Crowdfunding for the UK National Health Service. *Social Science & Medicine*, 308, 115214. Retrieved from https://doi.org/10.1016/j.socscimed.2022.115214

Stone, Deborah. (2020). *Counting: How We Use Numbers to Decide What Matters*. New York: Liveright Publishing.

Stone, Diane. (1996). *Capturing the Political Imagination: Think Tanks and the Policy Process*. London: Routledge. Retrieved from https://doi.org/10.4324/9780203044292

Stoye, G. (2018). *NHS at 70: Does the NHS Need More Money and How Could We Pay for It?* London: Health Foundation. Retrieved from https://www.health.org.uk/publications/nhs-at-70-does-the-nhs-need-more-money-and-how-could-we-pay-for-it

Stuart, J., Kamerāde, D., Connolly, S., Paine, A. E., Nichols, G. and Grotz, J. (2020). *The Impacts of Volunteering on the Subjective Wellbeing of Volunteers: A Rapid Evidence Assessment*. London: What Works Centre for Wellbeing.

Sturdy, S. (2002). *Medicine, Health and the Public Sphere in Britain, 1600–2000*. London: Routledge.

Tavares, S., Proença, T. and Ferreira, M. R. (2022). The Challenges of Formal Volunteering in Hospitals. *Health Services Management Research*, 35(2), 114–126. Retrieved from https://doi.org/10.1177/09514848211010255

Taylor, H. (2022, 17 April). Volunteers to Be Used for 999 Calls in London as Ambulance Service Struggles. *The Guardian*. Retrieved from https://www.theguardian.com/society/2022/apr/18/volunteers-to-be-used-for-999-calls-in-london-as-ambulance-service-struggles

The Health Foundation. (2018). NHS at 70: Public Perceptions. Retrieved from https://health.org.uk/publications/reports/nhs-at-70-public-perceptions

The Health Foundation. (2022) Public Perceptions of the NHS and Social Care: Performance, Policy and Expectations. Retrieved from https://www.health.org.uk/publications/long-reads/public-perceptions-performance-policy-and-expectations

The Health Foundation and Ipsos. (2022a). Public Perceptions of Health and Social Care (November–December 2021). London: The Health Foundation. Retrieved from https://www.health.org.uk/publications/public-perceptions-of-health-and-social-care-november-december-2021

The Health Foundation and Ipsos. (2022b). Public Perceptions of Health and Social Care (May–June 2022). London: The Health Foundation. Retrieved from https://www.health.org.uk/publications/public-perceptions-of-health-and-social-care-wave-2-may-june-2022

The King's Fund. (2022). Key Facts and Figures About the NHS. Retrieved from https://www.kingsfund.org.uk/audio-video/key-facts-figures-nhs

Thomson, M. (2021). Branding. Retrieved from https://peopleshistorynhs.org/encyclopaedia/branding/

Thomson, M. (2022). Representation of the NHS in the Arts and Popular Culture. In J. Crane and J. Hand (Eds), *Posters, Protests, and Prescriptions: Cultural Histories of the National Health Service in Britain*. Manchester: Manchester University Press.

Thorlby, R., Gardner, T. and Turton, C. (2019). *NHS Performance and Waiting Times* (p 15). London: The Health Foundation. Retrieved from https://www.health.org.uk/sites/default/files/2019-11/nhs-performance-and-waiting-times-priorities-for-the-next-government-ge02-.pdf

Tichenor, M., Merry, S. E., Grek, S. and Bandola-Gill, J. (2022). Global Public Policy in a Quantified World: Sustainable Development Goals as Epistemic Infrastructures. *Policy and Society* 41(4), 431–444.

Tierney, S. and Mahtani, K. (2020, April 23). Volunteering During the COVID-19 Pandemic: What Are the Potential Benefits to People's Well-being. Retrieved from https://socialprescribing.phc.ox.ac.uk/news-views/views/volunteering-during-the-covid-19-pandemic-what-are-the-potential-benefits-to-people2019s-well-being

Tierney, S., Wong, G., Roberts, N., Boylan, A.-M., Park, S., Abrams, R. et al (2020). Supporting Social Prescribing in Primary Care by Linking People to Local Assets: A Realist Review. *BMC Medicine*, 18(1), 49. Retrieved from https://doi.org/10.1186/s12916-020-1510-7

Titmuss, R. M. (2004). *Private Complaints and Public Health: Richard Titmuss on the National Health Service*. Bristol: Policy Press.

Tuohy, Carolyn H. (2019). The National Health Service (NHS) at 70: Some Comparative Reflections. *Health Economics, Policy and Law*, 14(1), 25–28. Retrieved from https://doi.org/10.1017/S1744133118000105

Tuohy, C. H. (2023). Anniversary Narratives of the Healthcare State: Institutional Entrenchment in Retrospect. *Journal of Health Politics, Policy and Law*, 48(2). Retrieved from https://doi.org/10.1215/03616878-10234212

Vindrola-Padros, C. and Whiteford, L. M. (2021). Comparative Health Systems: Paradigm Changes. In S. C. Scrimshaw, S. D. Lane, R. A. Rubinstein and J. Fisher (Eds), *The SAGE Handbook of Social Studies in Health and Medicine* (2nd edn) (pp 359–372). London: SAGE.

Voß, J.-P. and Freeman, R. (2015). *Knowing Governance: The Epistemic Construction of Political Order*. Basingstoke: Palgrave Macmillan.

Vote Leave. (2015). Briefing: The EU Is a Threat to the NHS. Retrieved from http://www.voteleavetakecontrol.org/briefing_health

Vote Leave. (2016). NHS 6 page leaflet. Retrieved from https://d3n8a8pro7vhmx.cloudfront.net/voteleave/pages/2318/attachments/original/1458064107/NEW_A5_NHS_6_page_leaflet_PRINT_NEW.pdf?1458064107

Warnes, W. (2022, 1 August). St John Crews to Drive 999 Ambulances. *East Anglian Daily Times*. Retrieved from https://www.eadt.co.uk/news/health/st-johns-ambulance-crews-to-drive-999-ambulances-9181456

Weale, A. (2015). Reflecting on 'Are Health Problems Systemic? Politics of Access and Choice under Beveridge and Bismarck Systems'. *Health Economics, Policy and Law*, 10(4), 431–435. Retrieved from https://doi.org/10.1017/S1744133115000171

Webster, C. (2002). *National Health Service: A Political History* (2nd edn). Oxford: Oxford University Press.

Wellings, D. (2022, 26 October). Has the Public Fallen Out of Love with the NHS? Retrieved from https://www.kingsfund.org.uk/blog/2022/10/has-public-fallen-out-love-nhs

Wellings, D., Jefferies, D., Maguire, D., Appleby, J., Hemmings, N., Morris, J. and Schlepper, L. (2022). Public Satisfaction with the NHS and Social Care in 2021: Results from the British Social Attitudes Survey. London: The King's Fund and Nuffield Trust. Retrieved from https://www.nuffieldtrust.org.uk/files/2022-03/bsa-survey-report-2nd-pp.pdf

Wendt, C., Kohl, J., Mischke, M. and Pfeifer, M. (2010). How Do Europeans Perceive Their Healthcare System? Patterns of Satisfaction and Preference for State Involvement in the Field of Healthcare. *European Sociological Review*, 26(2), 177–192.

Wendt, C., Mischke, M. and Pfeifer, M. (2011). *Welfare States and Public Opinion: Perceptions of Healthcare Systems, Family Policy and Benefits for the Unemployed and Poor in Europe*. Cheltenham: Edward Elgar Publishing.

Williams, W. (2020). *Windrush Lessons Learned Review: Independent Review*. Home Office. Retrieved from https://www.gov.uk/government/publications/windrush-lessons-learned-review

Woodhead, C., Stoll, N., Harwood, H., Team, T. S., Alexis, O. and Hatch, S. L. (2022). 'They Created a Team of Almost Entirely the People Who Work and Are Like Them': A Qualitative Study of Organisational Culture and Racialised Inequalities among Healthcare Staff. *Sociology of Health & Illness*, 44(2), 267–289. Retrieved from https://doi.org/10.1111/1467-9566.13414

Wynne, B. (2006). Public Engagement as a Means of Restoring Public Trust in Science: Hitting the Notes, But Missing the Music? *Public Health Genomics*, 9(3), 211–220.

Young, I., Davis, M., Flowers, P. and McDaid, L. M. (2019). Navigating HIV Citizenship: Identities, Risks and Biological Citizenship in the Treatment as Prevention Era. *Health, Risk & Society*, 21(1–2), 1–16. Retrieved from https://doi.org/10.1080/13698575.2019.1572869

Young, P. (2011, 5 April). NatCen Social Research. Retrieved from https://www.natcen.ac.uk/blog/putting-public-satisfaction-and-patient-experience-at-the-heart-of-the-nhs

Younge, G. (2020, 5 May). Gary Younge: What, Precisely, Are We Making Noise For?. *Financial Times*. Retrieved from https://www.ft.com/content/185dd664-83da-11ea-b6e9-a94cffd1d9bf

Younge, G. (2022, 23 March). What Does it Mean to Be British? *The New Statesman*. Retrieved from https://www.newstatesman.com/politics/a-dream-of-britain/2022/03/what-does-it-mean-to-be-british

Index

References to figures appear in *italic* type; those in **bold** type refer to tables.

Printed and bound by CPI Group (UK) Ltd, Croydon, CR0 4YY

16/04/2025

14658341-0005